Photographs by Alexandria Mauck
Cover design by Mary Kate Murphy
Book design by Eric Schall

ISBN-13: 978-0-9860915-1-3

This book is intended to serve as a reference and is not intended to be used as a medical manual. The information is not intended to replace the advice of a doctor. PreTrain, LLC disclaims any liability for the decisions you make based on the information present. If you suspect that you have a medical problem, we urge you to seek competent medical help.

The information in this book is meant to complement a proper exercise and health program. It is not intended to replace or substitute any exercise routine prescribed by your doctor. The editors of PreTrain advise readers to take full responsibility for their health, their safety, and to not take risks beyond your level of experience, training, or current fitness level. As with all exercise programs, you should get your doctor's approval before beginning.

Mentioning of specific companies, organizations, or authorities in this book does not imply endorsement by the author, nor does mention of specific companies, organization or authorities imply that they endorse this book, its author, or the publisher.

PreTrain Fundamentals

6 WEEKS TO A STRONG, STABLE, AND FLEXIBLE BODY

Camilla Moore, D.C.

Feel free to move for the rest of your life.

Dedication

This work is dedicated to my family. To Mom and Dad, you are the best people I know. All the sacrifices you made for us in so many ways, I want you to know it was worth it. I couldn't have done this without the lessons we learned. You taught us to believe in ourselves and it started with you believing in us. Most of all, I am thankful you showed us what it means to be a good person. I hope we have made you proud. To my sisters, Ange and Vaness, I am thankful for our friendship every day, and am so grateful we have each other as sisters.

This program is dedicated to my patients. You are an inspiration every day.

And for my little family of Jake and Jack - never have I had such fullness in my heart. Your love, happiness, and laughter makes every day better than the last. Jake, you have redefined partnership for me. You are my New Year.

Gratitude

A heartfelt thank you goes to Crystal Milligan and Adriana Ferns for your perspectives and training expertise.

Thank you to Chelsey and Karen, two wonderful people. Your dedication and commitment to your work has helped make this possible.

Thank you to our amazing video models Peter Holland and Lizzie Newton. You made our production day so wonderful and I appreciate your hard work preparing for it.

To my sweet friend and tireless supporter, Blaine Hudson, you are amongst the kindest souls I have met.

To my amazing rock stars: Mary Kate Murphy, Diane Sterrett, and Sara. Thank you for making this experience a positive and collective success, and thank you for being extraordinary at what you do.

A deep thank you goes to my focus group for dedicating time, effort, and invaluable feedback. A special thank you to Scott. You are an inspiration and I will be forever grateful and touched that you allowed me to be a part of your journey.

Gratitude also goes to out to the guys at All the Way Around: Chandler, Peter, Scott, and Kevin. Thank you for an amazing experience.

No provider or heath care practitioner would be where we are today without the works of individuals that came before us. We owe it to them, to our present patients, and to the future of medicine, to question that which we know, to explore that which we think, and to trust that which we feel. Thank you to those whose works have led us to this point, and thank you to those who continue to push our limits to see what is possible.

Table of Contents

Introduction

At PreTrain, we believe that the best fitness routine is the one that works best for you and that you can keep up long term. PreTrain is an approach to health that focuses on moving right so you can move more and move well. It teaches proper movement that minimizes the risk of injury, built on the idea that fitness and training should make you healthier and stronger, not cause injury.

As a chiropractor who focuses on assessing patient movement, I have found that most injuries are caused by an imbalance in the stability, strength and flexibility of muscles. Some muscle groups become overworked and injured, while others become underworked and weak. I developed the PreTrain series of exercises to target the most common areas of imbalance and the muscles that you use every day, applied with an educated and holistic approach to fitness.

PreTrain Fundamentals is the first step-by-step instructional program that targets proper movement patterns and focuses on three main pillars of fitness: strength, stability, and flexibility. In doing so, PreTrain answers a broad spectrum of fitness questions including:

Where do I start with an exercise program?
What exercises do I need to do to minimize the risk of repetitive use injuries?
How do I transition from one type of training program to another?
How do I complement my existing training program to reduce my risk of injury?
I have finished treatment for an injury. Now what?
How do I return to fitness after having my baby?

Whether it is riding your bike, training for a triathlon, or lifting up your grandchildren, PreTrain can help you do the things that are important to you.

PART
1

How It All Began

"Feed the soil, and let the soil feed the plant."

PreTrain is rooted in a holistic approach

I was raised in rural Maine on vegetables grown in our garden, grass fed beef pastured in our fields, and honey spun from Dad's beehives. Organic was not a label, it was a way of life. As it turns out, we were cool and hip before catchphrases like "Organic" or "Farm to Table" became cool and hip. We had fulfillment in three main aspects of our life: physical health, spiritual health, and emotional health. My dad loved his organic gardens and lived by the sustainability motto, "Feed the soil and let the soil feed the plant." I have found success by applying those early balance lessons to every aspect of my life, including patient care.

When I began my chiropractic practice in 2008 I decided to specialize in athletic injuries, specifically overuse injuries to the low back, hip, shoulder, knee and ankle. I have found no shortage of patients. These injuries were not difficult to treat if the evaluation was thorough and the treatment was appropriate for the diagnosis. However, I would see patients in my office with the same injury time and time again. How could this be? Hadn't we fixed this the first time? It became obvious that the treatment, though appropriate and effective, was not enough. The treatment alone was not sustainable.

After working with several offices in Southern New England, I opened my own practice in Bristol, RI within a well-utilized fitness facility. Many of my new patients were gym members and, with their permission, I began collaborating with their personal trainers throughout their treatment plans for a comprehensive approach. I also adapted my evaluations to include an assessment of three key areas of the patient's general fitness: flexibility, stability, and strength.

> 1. Flexibility: We addressed flexibility issues of the joints and muscles, mobilizing tightened, overworked, and injured muscles.
> 2. Stability: We provided targeted, rehabilitative exercises to stabilize and reset the affected areas.
> 3. Strength: We created specific strengthening programs to encourage balanced and coordinated muscle development.

The results were dynamic.

We were resolving injuries in half the time and patients were lifting heavier weights, running faster, and training longer. Most importantly, however, the combination of flexibility, stability, and strength training was providing a long-term solution for injuries that had often plagued patients for years. The exercises prescribed initially served to target specific areas based on my evaluation of their condition. We mobilized what was restricted, stabilized what was unstable, and strengthened what was weak. It took daily attention and work, but after a few weeks, these exercises served to complement their existing exercise program rather than define or replace them. The rehabilitative exercises initially taught then served as "maintenance" exercises that could be performed on a regular but infrequent basis to prevent their injuries from returning or recurring. By focusing on those three functional pillars of fitness, we had developed a more sustainable model of fitness for everyday athletes.

Another change I made to my Bristol practice model was to increase the amount of treatment time for each visit. Having my own practice gave me the welcome opportunity to simplify, lowering the high patient volume required at other clinics and lengthening treatment sessions. I could spend more time evaluating and treating, and less time controlling the chaos of high volume. The result was more effective treatment and, most importantly, the opportunity to have truly open and honest conversations with patients. And as my patients spoke, I listened.

Patient dynamics led the way

Most patients came to me with the typical repetitive use injuries. They ranged from elite athletes to those with injuries from life's daily athletics and everyone in between. Hip pain, low back pain, shoulder pain, knee and ankle injuries were most common, and the standard approach was to recommend a core exercise program. The problem was that everyone was offering core exercises, which had become a staple in workout programs from boot camps to the self-created exercise programs. But not all core programs are created equal.

A strong and stable core is unquestionably important to overall wellness and fitness, but a fundamental question remained: If everyone was doing core exercises, why were they still getting overuse injuries that had overt core weakness as a key component? Why, in functional tests performed during my examination, were they unable to stabilize their pelvis and low back with even the slightest amount of stress? *Why were these core exercises ineffective?*

It was clear that a lack of effort was not the culprit: these patients were working their core in a dozen different ways on a dozen different days. Something was obviously missing from their exercise and training routines. I began digging deeper into their medical history, specifically their history of injuries and past trauma, searching for the answer that I eventually uncovered.

Many of my patients had been active on some level, at some point, for most of their life. Although they were aware of the obvious changes that accompany time and age, such as changes in their posture and the presence of new aches and pains, patients were unaware of how these changes affected the way they moved on a day to day basis. They didn't realize their overuse injuries today were a direct result of physical changes from their past. Those old injuries had resulted in compensations and adaptations that made it difficult to actually activate the deep muscles of the core.

Patients were physically able to perform the exercises; however, they were simply using their bigger muscles to move rather than using the deep core muscles underneath. Compensating in this way led to improper movement – which is why PreTrain focuses on building a foundation of proper movement on three pillars: Stability, Flexibility, and Strength.

When we applied this three-tiered approach, we not only successfully treated acute injuries, patients reported improvements in secondary issues such as chronic muscle tightness and other nagging injuries.

The need was clear, and I knew I needed to share the solution we'd developed. PreTrain Fundamentals was born.

How PreTrain Fundamentals retrains your movement

PreTrain Fundamentals is designed to teach and educate, so you learn **how** your body should move. You'll learn to feel the difference between proper movement patterns, and the ones you have fallen into over a lifetime of everyday movement. PreTrain's approach is to offer corrective exercises that train your body to be comfortable and strong in the correct pattern of movement.

PreTrain focuses on building flexible and stable parts. Then, we coordinate the parts to move as a whole. Finally, we add a short-duration, high intensity training program that will strengthen and build the muscle to support these movements, locking in your new movement pattern with your own strength. **The result: strong, sustainable bodies that can adapt to any of life's physical challenges.**

But before we get into specifics, it's helpful to look at how we move.

"Let's make sure we are moving correctly, before we move faster, longer, and in more complicated ways."

How we move and how we end up moving wrong

We all have one ideal way of moving. The actual way you move is based on many factors, starting with genetic makeup. Just as we inherit facial features, height, and weight, the more subtle body and posture features are also inherited. The body's function, or the way we move, is based on the structure, or what we look like on the inside.

A look at the inside:

Joints – Joints are the hinges that move us. We have joints throughout our body from our toes to our head. Each joint is supposed to move a certain amount, in a certain way, to perform a certain function. For example, in order to bend down and touch our toes, each vertebra in our back has to move a little bit in order for our whole spine to move together.

Ligaments – Ligaments hold joints together, limit how much a joint can move and control the direction of that movement. Ligaments look like fiberglass tape wrapped around a joint in all directions, creating a protective capsule.

Muscles – Muscles provide the power that moves the joints. Like ligaments, muscles can limit and control the amount of movement of joints to an extent. However, unlike ligaments, we can strengthen muscles and therefore control how *well* they work. Some muscles, like the quadriceps muscle in the front of the thigh, are big and powerful. Other muscles, like the small multifidi in the spine, work to hold joints stable. In general, the smaller and closer to our skeleton the muscles are, the more they work to stabilize our skeleton when we move, thus protecting us from injury. The bigger "outer" muscles work to power us through our movements. The more stable we make the muscles with PreTrain, the more we are protected from injury.

Tendons – Tendons connect muscles to bones. They are like rubber bands that help control the connection between the joint and the muscle.

As we mentioned above, our movement pattern begins with our genes and how we're built. "*My whole family has bad backs*," is a phrase I often hear in the office. There isn't necessarily a bad back gene, but familial traits in our makeup may predispose us to certain injuries. Over time, your body goes through changes that may alter the underlying structure and, consequently, how you move. Recent studies indicate that movement not only changes after an injury, but the effects on movement can be seen throughout the whole body as the body adapts and compensates.

Therefore, the absence of pain does not necessarily mean an absence of injury or dysfunction.[1]

As an example, one of the most common old injuries my patients report is sprained ankles. Something seemingly trivial still changes the way we move while the ankle heals and the body changes. A temporary limp indicates that the unaffected side of the body is *working harder*, while the injured side *works less*. This imbalance may remain present unless it is treated with rehabilitation exercises, and can cause more significant problems down the road. In other words, pain can alter movement, but movement might remain altered even after the pain is resolved.

Regardless of individual movement patterns, there are certain areas of our bodies that need to be stable, others that need mobility and flexibility, and others that need to be strong.

The role of flexibility and mobility

Mobility describes how easily we move overall. Flexibility describes how easily our muscles move. PreTrain addresses both.

Flexibility in muscles is important; however, there are other structures that need to move as well. Joint mobility is equally as important. Mobility of the fascia, the connective tissue that weaves through our whole body and keeps us together, is also necessary for fluid movement and injury prevention. Flexibility and mobility are necessary to create room for movement. The more flexible and mobile our body is, the better it can handle a demand placed on that body. Think about it in terms of your daily schedule: The more flexible the time in your day, the more you are able to adapt to changes that may occur during that day. The same is true for our body.

Many people think their muscles are too tight: *"My hamstrings are always tight, even though I stretch them every day."* This is a common complaint I hear in the office. However, if the problem is a tight hamstring, and the solution to tight hamstrings is to stretch them, then shouldn't the result be a more flexible hamstring? Shouldn't you see the results?

But there's more to it than simply stretching.

When muscles become overworked, the restriction is not just from a shortening (tightening) of the muscle, but also from scar tissue that builds up within the muscle. Constant tension on muscles will result in increased friction and tension within the muscle fibers. This leads to less blood flow and scar tissue is formed in between the fascial sheath of the muscle fibers. This creates adhesions, affectionately referred to as "gunk," that will restrict the movement of the muscle as a whole, leaving you with the feeling of tightness such as tight hamstrings.

Progressive therapies that chiropractors, physical therapists and massage therapists use (such as myofascial release techniques) work to break up these adhesions, freeing them up to allow more mobility in the muscle. The result is more specific flexibility and therefore more global mobility. At home, foam rolling is one of the most effective and versatile home remedies to achieve similar results. PreTrain uses the foam roller to more gently break up these adhesions, followed by stretching to lengthen the muscles and fascia. That's just one more way PreTrain is so much more than a fitness routine.

Recall that muscles function properly when they are at their proper length. Now think of power. A muscle and joint complex that is able to move within its full range of motion has more power. It has the ability to be stronger.

The role of stability

If some muscles are restricted, tight, and overworked, the next logical inquiry is to determine which muscles are *under*worked. This leads to the topic of stability and the role of the muscles that stabilize our body.

The muscles that stabilize our body are the deepest muscles in our body. They live closest to our bones and protect us from injury. Like a high-rise building's steel frame, a strong and stable foundation is paramount to a fit body. Stabilizing muscles control your body's ability to balance. Therefore, stability and balance are necessarily interconnected. To improve balance, you must improve stability, and by improving stability, you can improve balance. A stable foundation also allows the other, bigger muscle groups to have a solid base from which to power.

The deep muscles that work to stabilize and protect your body are difficult to target with full body exercise, they require very focused and isolated exercises, often referred to as rehabilitation exercises. These are usually reserved for office visits at the chiropractor or physical therapist, but you get them through PreTrain, professionally demonstrated and executed as if you were at an office visit.

When the stabilizing muscles become weak, the bigger and stronger muscles are called into service to compensate. An overworked larger muscle, doing double duty to provide stability, quickly reaches a breaking point, causing pain and injury. At this point, two issues need to be addressed:

(1) the muscles that are injured; and
(2) the weak muscles that started the chain reaction.

PreTrain Fundamentals begins with these targeted core exercises. The concept is to first target common areas of weakness in the deep stabilizing muscles, and then build flexibility, mobility, and strength around a foundation of properly functioning stabilizing muscles. Many people use term "core" to refer to the muscles within our low back and pelvis that protect our low back. This group of deep stabilizing muscles are at the center of your body, and are very important. However, this core is just one set of stabilizing muscles within your body.

You have a similar core throughout the foot and ankle, hips, back, and shoulders, just as a high-rise building has steel girders from foundation to rooftop. Think of all your core muscles as the protective muscles that protect each joint throughout your body.

The role of strength

Strength training is the most common component of any fitness program. PreTrain takes a unique approach to strength by focusing on strengthening the small, deep stabilizing muscles first, before building strength in the bigger muscle groups. Strength training in the bigger muscle groups is limited by stability from the small stabilizing muscles and overall flexibility. Too often, people bypass building a foundation of flexibility and stability, and try to just strengthen the bigger (more visible) muscles. This unbalanced (unstable) focus on strength is what often leads to overworked muscles, pain, and injury.

Strength training is vital to improve muscle quality, and is an appropriate aspect for each and every fitness regime. The exercises in *Module 3: Excel* of PreTrain Fundamentals focus on strengthening the small stabilizing muscles in conjunction with the bigger muscle groups. Training tools such as the Bosu ball allow for complex exercises that will build strength in the stabilizing muscles and challenge the bigger muscles, ultimately leading to a powerful combination of strength and stability.

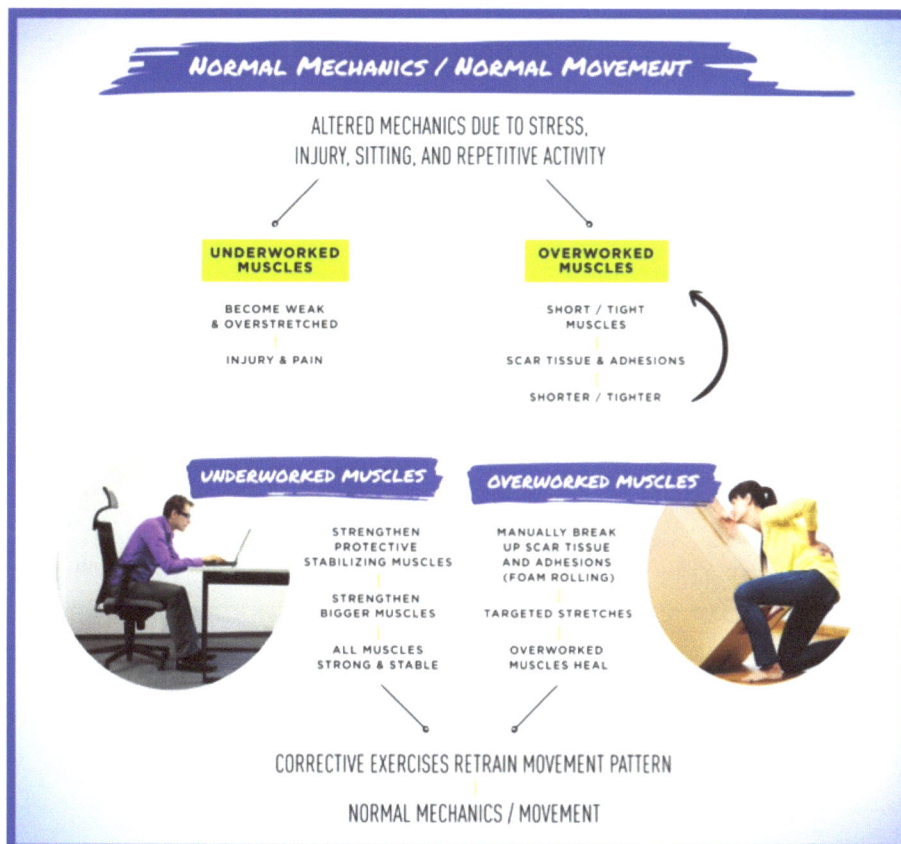

Chapter 3 - The Program

"Rethink your body."

Three Modules help retrain your body

PreTrain Fundamentals starts with the basics and then builds with three distinctive modules. Each module builds on the progress from the previous set of exercises. Within each module there are two levels of increasing difficulty. The modules are designed to be completed in order, and each level should be mastered before graduating to the next module. It is important to note that, although each level is intended to provide one week of daily exercises, your ability to maintain form throughout the proscribed number of repetitions should determine your readiness for the next level or module.

PreTrain Basics walks you through the three unique features of PreTrain Fundamentals: The PreTrain Brace, the Shoulder Brace, and the Lower Extremity Brace. These three fundamental movements begin with proper breathing and correlate how to engage, or activate, the most important stabilizing muscles in your body. These three Braces will be applied to exercises throughout the program.

Module 1: Rebuild. This focuses on the most basic movements, and the most commonly weak muscles. We apply the PreTrain Brace and Shoulder Brace to isolate the small, deep stabilizing muscles of your core and shoulders and to rebuild stability lost over time.

Module 2: Restore. This incorporates the stability work from Module 1 into weight bearing exercises that promote proper movement and control, and includes mobility and flexibility. You will learn how to squat correctly, how to move through your hips rather than your back, all while strengthening the big muscle groups in your body. Module 2 also provides instruction on how to engage the small, stabilizing muscles of the foot and ankle while restoring your body's ability to coordinate movement together as a whole unit.

Module 3: Excel. This is a high-intensity, short duration, functional workout. Module 3 builds on the skills mastered in Modules 1 and 2 to strengthen and train your body in your new way of moving. It will get your heart rate up and your metabolism rockin', while focusing on form and quality rather than quantity. Module 3 is meant to build overall strength and endurance for life, giving you the tools to excel at whatever you chose. Let's go!

	Module 1: Rebuild	Module 2: Restore	Module 3: Excel
Intensive, isolated core stability training	●		
Shoulder strengthening	●	●	●
Hip and low back strengthening	●	●	●
Advanced core stability applied to everyday movements		●	●
Advanced balance training		●	●
Foot and ankle strengthening		●	●
Intermediate core stability		●	
Flexibility training to protect joints and muscles		●	
Overall mobility training		●	
Beginnning balance training		●	
Movement training		●	
Introduction to functional training			●
Advanced functional training			●

NOTE: we created PreTrain Fundamentals in multiple media formats (DVD, streaming, eBook) to respond to individual learning styles. You advance at your pace in the way that works best for you.

How to use PreTrain Fundamentals

First and foremost, PreTrain Fundamentals has limitations. It was developed to address the most common issues we have noticed in most people. It does not address all issues for all people. As a clinician, I believe nothing replaces a one-on-one evaluation with a trained health care professional: your physician, your physical therapist, your chiropractor, or a specialist. This program is a functional program and if something does not feel right, the appropriate response is a functional evaluation. Not sure? Just ask your health care provider.

PreTrain Fundamentals was designed to improve the way you move on a daily basis. It is accessible and effective, limiting the time to 20 minutes per day, and can be performed at the gym, at home, or in the park – it goes where you go. It serves to complement your existing training program, as an extension of a physical rehabilitation program, or a beginning step to transition into a new or different exercise program.

PreTrain can be completed in as little as six weeks, but it is designed so you can move at a pace that is specific and comfortable to you. You may move through the entire *Module 1: Rebuild* in two weeks. Or it may take you four weeks just to master the first level of *Module 1: Rebuild*. That's okay! You move at your own pace, this is not a competition. Practice it. Work through it. Master it. Become empowered. Approach these exercises as tests that you perform each day, getting you ready for the next challenge life throws your way, whether it's lifting a grocery bag, weeding the garden, or climbing the stairs.

Training the core

Here's an interesting question: Is it possible to have a routine full of core exercises and still have a weak core? Absolutely! It is entirely (and frequently) possible to perform an exercise using the wrong muscles. The plank (a great exercise to maintain and strengthen the core muscles) is a good example of a core exercise many people perform improperly. Without an understanding of which muscles to use, and if the core muscles have not been adequately trained, the other, bigger and more superficial muscles in the back and hips will take over. So even though you can maintain the plank position, you won't be strengthening the deep stabilizing muscles.

In PreTrain Basics, we spend vital time teaching the basic methods for engaging these deep muscles, which are then strengthened in *Module 1: Rebuild*, before we move into an advanced exercise such as the plank in *Module 3: Excel*.

Remember those deep, stabilizing muscles throughout the whole body? PreTrain Basics addresses each of these in three different areas: the lower extremity (foot, ankle, knee, hip), the upper extremity (shoulders and upper back), and the low back and pelvis.

Stability and balance are actually a result of the interconnected network of stabilizing muscles from your toes to your head, beginning with the muscles of the foot and ankle. When you walk, small muscles in your foot and lower leg are engaged to begin the stability pathway, which continues up your leg, into your hip, and into your core. Therefore, the stability of your core is only as strong as the stability of your hip. The stability of your hip is only as strong as the stability of your knee. The stability of your knee is only as strong as the stability of your foot and ankle. And the stability of your foot and ankle is only as strong as the muscles within it. These muscles are most challenged with bare feet. Therefore, in a program where we are working to improve and maximize stability, it is important to challenge the beginning of the stability chain in the foot and ankle muscles.

A word about footwear.

Stability prevents injury and protects us when we move, and shoes supplement our body's natural ability to stabilize, which provides a strong basis from which to move.

To maximize the ability to stabilize your core, your footwear should be minimal to encourage the stabilizing muscles in your lower extremities to work the hardest. The appropriate footwear is different for everyone. Start with a stable sneaker that you feel comfortable wearing. As your strength and stability improve, you may be able to change to a less stable shoe, and move on to bare feet. Don't hesitate to check in with your physical therapist, podiatrist, orthopedist, or functional chiropractor with any questions on deciding which shoes are most appropriate for you.

Your core is more complex than you think

PreTrain Fundamentals begins with non-weight bearing stabilizing exercises to isolate the core muscles without being limited by the stability of the joints below it. You'll learn how to stabilize just the core complex without the added difficulty of the stabilizing chain from the foot and ankle, and all the way up.

We start by teaching proper breathing technique. Your diaphragm is the top of the core complex. It provides stability to the spine, support for the lungs, and serves as an important conduit for blood vessels and nerves. Many people breath through their chest rather than their diaphragm. This is a common adaptation resulting from prolonged sitting, desk work, and increased stress. Simply breathing incorrectly can lead to a loss of stability, to which the diaphragm is intended to contribute.

Second, we learn how to activate the diaphragm with the pelvic floor. The pelvic floor provides support from the bottom and creates a sling for the organs. Third, we learn how to activate the transversus abdominus that stabilizes the core complex on the side.

Finally, we learn how to activate the deep, small muscles in the back that support the spine. Together, these four groups of muscles create the core group of muscles, which provide the underlying foundation for stability. We eventually work into weight-bearing exercises, to include stability in the whole body from the foot to the neck.

The PreTrain Edge

We cannot eliminate injuries. However, in my experience, there is a lot that can be done to minimize the possibility, and mitigate the severity, of injuries. In order to do so, we must start with the fundamentals. Your mindset needs to be one of building knowledge, building strength, and building sustainability by starting small. We often put great emphasis on **looking** fit and healthy that we often forget to actually **be** fit and healthy. It's a fundamental paradigm shift.

PreTrain Fundamentals is about returning to the basics of health and wellness by focusing on the fundamentals of movement, to attain fitness through improving mobility, stability, and strength, one solid step at time, and give you tools for a lifetime of good movement. Ready to get started?

P A R T
2

PreTrain Fundamentals

"Relearning movement is like learning another language. First, learn the alphabet. Then, make the words. Finally, make new sentences."

The PreTrain Basics are four specific "moves" that are applied to exercises throughout the PreTrain program. They teach you how to "turn on" and use the most important stabilizing muscles in your body. The PreTrain Brace activates the complicated core muscles of the back and abdomen, the Shoulder Brace activates the muscles in the shoulders, and the Lower Extremity Brace activates the muscles of the foot and ankle, legs, and hips.

The PreTrain Brace is the foundation of every exercise in PreTrain Fundamentals. The PreTrain Brace activates the core complex and provides stability throughout the low back and pelvis. We define the core as having four distinctive elements:

1. The diaphragm (the roof of the core)

2. The pelvic floor (the floor of the core)

3. The transversus abdominis (the sidewalls of the core)

4. The multifidi (the back walls of the core)

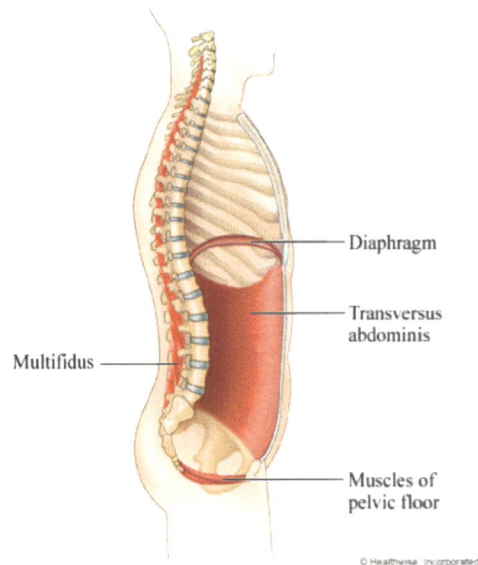

We will learn how to first engage the diaphragm (roof), then the pelvic floor (floor), then the transversus abdominis (sidewalls). Then, we will learn how to activate them together as a unit. This will create the PreTrain Brace. By mastering the PreTrain Brace and applying it to real life movements, you will be able to be stronger and more stable in each movement you make throughout the day. The multifidi (back walls) will be engaged throughout each exercise.

Hook-lying position

To learn how to activate all four parts of the PreTrain Brace, begin by lying on your back with your knees bent. Make sure your knees, feet, and hips are all in one line, and your low back is "neutral." Do not arch your back, do not flatten your back. To test, slip your flat hand under your back. Your back muscles should be relaxed as you find "your normal." If you can fit your hand and touch both your back and the floor, this is your neutral position.

1. The diaphragm (roof of core)

Located at the base of the lungs between the chest and abdominal cavity is the diaphragm, a dome shaped muscle which is the most efficient muscle of breathing. As the diaphragm contracts, the volume of the rib cage increases and air is drawn into the lungs, aided by the intercostal muscles.

Throughout the floor exercises, remember to breathe and breathe correctly! Most people breathe through their chest, a product of sitting for prolonged periods of time and a generally common, but physiologically abnormal, amount of emotional stress. By using the muscles in your chest to breathe, the diaphragm muscle may become weak. Because the diaphragm is a quarter of the core complex, weakness in the diaphragm muscle results in potential 25% loss of core stability.

To learn diaphragmatic breathing:
Lay on your back with your knees bent. Place one hand on your belly and one hand on your chest. Take a deep breath. How much does your top hand move? How much does your bottom hand move? Take a mental note.

Try breathing again. This time, focus on your ribcage expanding and your belly pushing out as you fill your lungs with air. Your bottom hand will push your belly out and your bottom hand will rise. Visualize your diaphragm dropping down in towards your abdomen. Take five deep belly breaths.

2. Pelvic floor (floor)

To activate the floor of the core complex, we will use a Kegel exercise. To identify the muscles in the pelvic floor, use the muscles you use to stop the stream of urination. These are very subtle contractions and can be performed without anyone noticing. Tighten these muscles and think of "lifting" the pelvic floor up towards your belly button. These muscles help to support the organs in your abdomen while providing support to the pelvic girdle. They are extremely important. Weakness in these muscles not only leads to instability within the pelvis, it can also cause complications such as incontinence and prolapse of the uterus or bladder.

Once you have found and activated these muscles, hold the contraction for five seconds. Relax for five seconds. Practice until you are able to contract the muscles for 10 seconds at a time.

3. Diaphragm and pelvic floor (roof plus floor)

Next, we are going to learn how to engage the roof and floor of the PreTrain Brace together. We are going to engage the diaphragm with the Kegel. To begin, take three deep belly breaths. Remember to feel the air expand your rib cage and fill your lungs, pushing your belly out as you breathe in. Let it relax as you breathe out. Next, perform a Kegel exercise to contract and lift the pelvic floor. Take another belly breath and as you breathe out, and lift the bottom of the pelvic floor up towards the belly button.

As you breathe in, let the pelvic floor drop and relax the muscles. As you breathe out, perform the Kegel, visualizing the pelvic floor lifting up towards your belly button.

Perform three sets of 10.

4. Diaphragm + pelvic floor + transversus abdominis (roof plus floor plus sidewalls)

We have learned how to engage the roof (diaphragm) and the floor (pelvic floor using a Kegel) of the core, and how to coordinate them together. The next step is to activate the sidewalls (the transversus abdominis, or TA, muscle).

To contract the TA, find the front of your hips, and place your thumbs on your hip   bones while allowing your fingertips to contact your belly. The contraction of the TA is very subtle. To perform, think of your belly as two different halves that meet in the middle at your belly button. Pull the halves together towards your belly button with your muscles. This will contract the TA. You will feel the contraction underneath your fingertips.

Now, let's add in the roof, floor, and put it all together.

Start with three deep belly breaths. Add in the Kegel. Perform three breaths, remembering to relax the pelvic floor while you inhale and contract the pelvic floor when you exhale.

Next, add in the TA contraction along with the Kegel. As you breathe in, relax both the Kegel and the TA. As you breathe out, contract the TA muscle and the Kegel together. This is the **PreTrain Brace**. Congratulations! You can now activate your entire core.

Quick review:

PreTrain Brace - Hook-lying position with spine in neutral. Knees, feet, hips all in one line.
- Deep breath to activate the diaphragm "roof"
- Kegel for pelvic floor "floor"
- Brace to activate "walls"
- Final breath while contracting PreTrain Brace

The bracing series is in PreTrain provide maximum stability within the joints. In his book, "Becoming a Supple Leopard," Dr. Kelly Starrett, explains how using torque, a normal force in physics, is not only advantageous when strengthen training, it is necessary for proper movement and preventing injury. Torque is the force generated in around an axis (ah yes, the high school physics is coming back to you!). In PreTrain, we refer to this as "locking in stability" with the PreTrain Brace, Shoulder Brace, and Lower Extremity Brace. These Braces are designed to create torque that protects joints and enhances the intention of each exercise.[2]

Shoulder Brace

The Shoulder Brace is used in conjunction with the PreTrain Brace. The Shoulder Brace engages the important stabilizing muscles of the shoulder and upper back. These muscles protect your neck, back, and shoulders. You can use the Shoulder Brace in a push up position, or in a standing position with rowing exercises.

1. Push up position
   a. Engage PreTrain Brace
   b. Place full palm of hand on the floor, feeling your whole hand contacting the floor.
   c. Feeling the weight of your body on the palm of your hand, with your hands secured, rotated your elbows to towards your side. Press your hand into the floor and attempt to turn your hand, without moving your hands, like you were going to open a jar that was stuck. Your elbows will rotate in towards your sides, but will remain straight.
   d. At the same time, you will feel your shoulder blades rotated back and down.
   e. Keep neck neutral and soft. This is the Shoulder Brace.

2. Row position
    a. Engage PreTrain Brace
    b. Holding your hands out in front of you with arms straight, rotated your shoulder blades back and down. You will feel the mid back muscles activate as your shoulder blades follow your shoulders back and down.

Lower Body Brace

The Lower Body Brace strengthens the small, stabilizing muscles in the foot and ankle, all the way up through the lower leg and into the thigh and hips. It is important to train these muscles as they need to work not only when we are exercising, but with every step we take.

    a. Engage PreTrain Brace
    b. Stand with feet 1 1/2 shoulder width apart. Pressing feet into the floor, feel the whole foot contact the floor.
    c. Press your feet into the floor and attempt to rotate your feet without moving them. Pretend you were trying to open a jar without moving your feet. You will feel all the muscles in your lower leg and hip engage. This is the Lower Body Brace.

Chapter 5 - Module 1: Rebuild

This series of exercises will help to rehabilitate the low back, hips, and shoulders.

Module 1: Rebuild has two levels of progression. Each level has a set of four exercises that should be performed successively. Each set should be repeated three times at least four times per week.

Module 1.1

All the exercises in Module 1, Level 1 work to strengthen the stabilizing muscles of the low back and pelvis while coordinating this stability with strength of the bigger muscle groups in the hip and back. Work at your own pace. This series of exercises are deceivingly difficult and may take a few weeks to master. Focus on maintaining stability throughout your low back and shoulders, and on keeping the PreTrain Brace and Shoulder Brace engaged throughout each exercise. This set of four exercises should be performed for three sets.

1. Bridging

A. Intention: This exercise begins to coordinate the PreTrain Brace, which connects your breathing and your core muscles, while building hip strength. The bridge series connects stabilizing muscles in the low back and pelvis with strength building power muscles in the hips. This coordination is important in preventing injury in the low back. The target hip muscle for this exercise is the gluteus maximus, or glute max. Throughout this exercise, focus on breathing out, contracting the PreTrain Brace, and activating your glute max all muscles at once.

B. Description: Lay on your back in the hook-lying position. Begin with the PreTrain Brace. Maintain the PreTrain Brace throughout the exercise, breathing normally but keeping the Kegel contracted. Keep your feet on the floor and as you lift up the hips, squeeze the glute max, and maintaining a 45 degree angle with your hips to the floor. Hold this for two seconds and lower your hips to the floor, controlling the movement. Perform 10 repetitions.

C. Common mistakes: Don't let the hips dip down when you come up into the bridge. Make sure you are lifting the hips up to a 45 degree angle and controlling the motion on the way down. You should feel the contraction in your glute max and not your hamstrings. If you hamstrings (the muscles in the back of your legs) cramp up, it is an indication your hamstring muscles are working harder than your glute max. This is counterproductive. Move your heels a little closer to your buttock to minimize the load on your hamstrings and isolate the glute max.

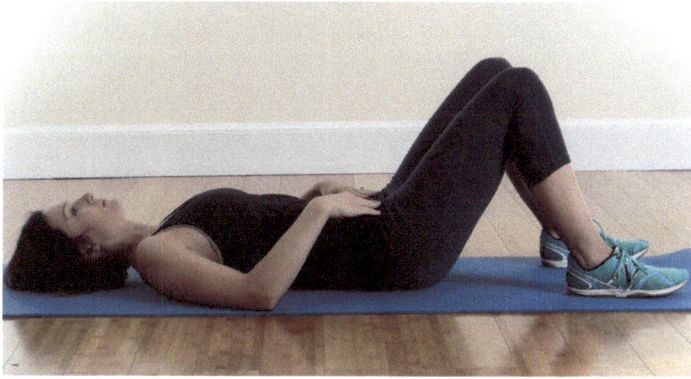

1A.
Lay on your back in a hook-lying position (knees, hips, and feet all in one line). Perform a PreTrain Brace.

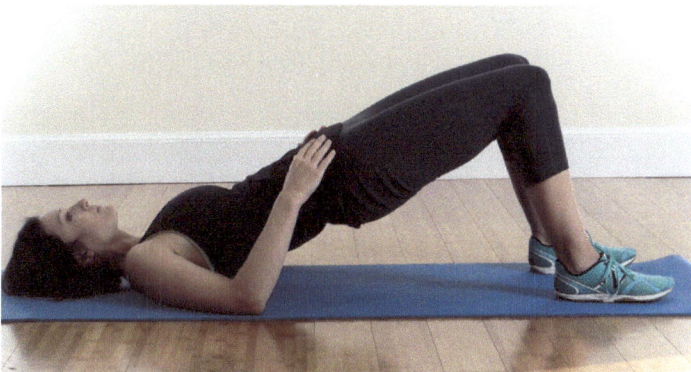

1B.
As you breathe out, squeeze your glutes and lift your hips up to make a 45 degree angle. If you feel tightness in your hamstrings, move your heels closer to your buttock to isolate the glute muscles even more.

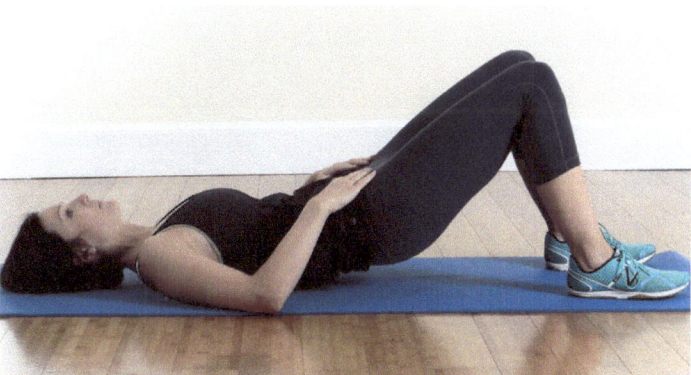

1C.
Common mistake. A common mistake is to not reach maximal hip extension, which will be less effective.

2. Dead Bug

A. Intention: This exercise begins to train your core, utilizing the PreTrain Brace, to be stable with movements that mimic every day walking and running. It begins to train "cross-body" stability that requires one side of your body to be stable while your opposite side moves.

B. Description: Begin with lying in a hook-lying position. Place palms of hands on the front of your hip bones. This will serve as a guide. Perform a PreTrain Brace. Maintaining the PreTrain Brace, lift one foot off the floor no more than 6 inches with a count of two seconds, and lower with a count of three seconds. The PreTrain Brace should hold your pelvis stable and your hips should not move. Alternate legs. Movements should be slow and steady. Perform 10 each side.

C. Common mistakes: Make sure your hips stay stable throughout the exercise, and that they do not move with leg movement. If you are having a hard time keeping your hips stable, as a temporary modification, you can press the opposite foot from the leg you are moving into the floor to recruit the glute max to help stabilize your pelvis. For example, if you are lifting your right foot, you can press your whole left foot into the floor to help. Be careful not to allow your left hip to rise off the floor. This is just a temporary modification. To move forward throughout the program, however, you must be able to stabilize you pelvis without this "help." Take your time with this exercise. It can be challenging for even the best conditioned athletes.

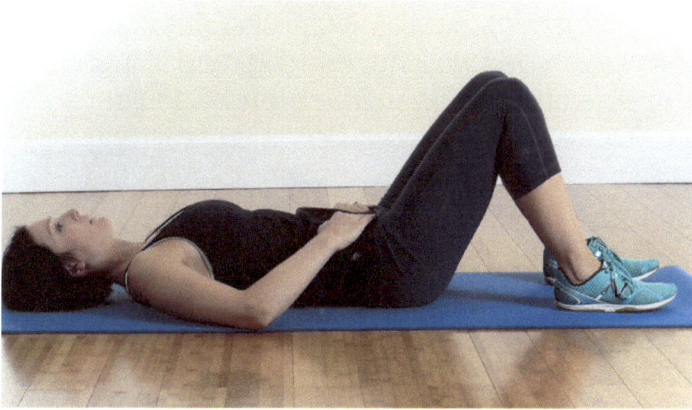

2A.
Start lying in a hook-lying position. Perform a PreTrain Brace.

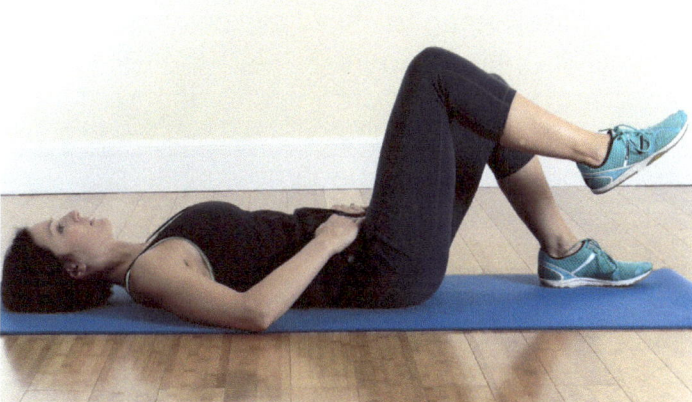

2B.
Keeping your PreTrain Brace engaged, slowly lift your foot off the floor. Keep your hands on your hip bones to serve as a guide. Your hands, and your hips, should stay stable.

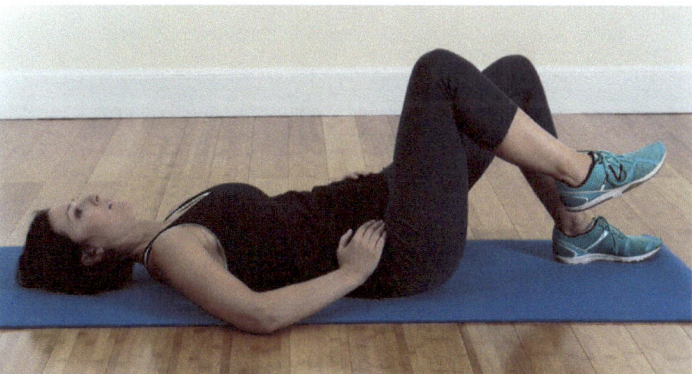

2C.
Common mistake: A common mistake is to not properly stabilize your core with the PreTrain Brace. You will see the right hip dip towards the floor as you life your right leg if your core is not properly engaged.

3. PreTrain Bird Dog

A. Intention: The PreTrain Bird Dog series is a modification of the Bird Dog exercise developed by Stuart McGill, PhD. This exercise focuses on stabilizing the core, pelvis, and shoulders in a way that mimics everyday walking, running, and lifting. The key to this exercise is maintaining a strong PreTrain Brace and Shoulder Brace throughout the whole exercise. This exercise strengthens the stabilizing muscles throughout the shoulder, low back, and pelvis while strengthening the bigger muscles that will help to support and move your body.

B. Description: Move to a quadruped position where you're on your hands and knees. Place your hands palm down on the floor and slightly wider than your shoulders. Your knees should be directly under your hips. Find the neutral spine position, without arching your flattening your back. Stabilize the pelvis and low back by performing a PreTrain Brace. To activate the shoulder girdle, perform the Shoulder Brace.

Once these muscles are engaged, slowly drag your right foot to straighten knee and squeeze the glutes, lifting the right leg until it is in line with your hip. Make sure your hips stay parallel to the floor and your right hip does not dip down as you contract your glute max. Keep your shoulders engaged. Slow and controlled, bend the knee and bring it back underneath your hip. Tap the knee to the floor. Keeping the knee bent, raise your leg out to the side no more than 30 degrees, feeling the muscle deep in the back of your hip contract. Make sure your back stays flat and spine neutral! Lower the leg until the knee is underneath your hip again.

Repeat with left leg.

After you have performed the exercise with the right leg, maintain your stability with the PreTrain Brace and Shoulder Brace. Slowly bring your right arm straight ahead of you with the thumb pointed to the ceiling. Feel the muscles in your back contract to lift your arm up. Bring the arm back down to the quadruped position. Tap the floor with your right hand. Bring your right arm out to the side, with the thumb pointed to the floor. Maintain stability with the PreTrain Brace and Shoulder Brace. Bring your right hand back down to the floor so it is under your shoulder. Repeat with left arm.

This series of exercises is repeated in the following order:
  Right arm forward
  Right arm to the side
  Left arm forward
  Left arm to the side
Right leg back
  Right leg to the side
  Left leg back
  Left leg to the side
  This series is repeated 5 times.

C. Common mistakes: Make sure to keep your hips level, your pelvis, low back, and upper back straight. Focus on squeezing your glute max to lift your leg. To modify, only lift your legs and your arms as far as you can while keeping your back straight. Work to get legs and arms in the same plane as your back, but take your time to get there in a correct way.

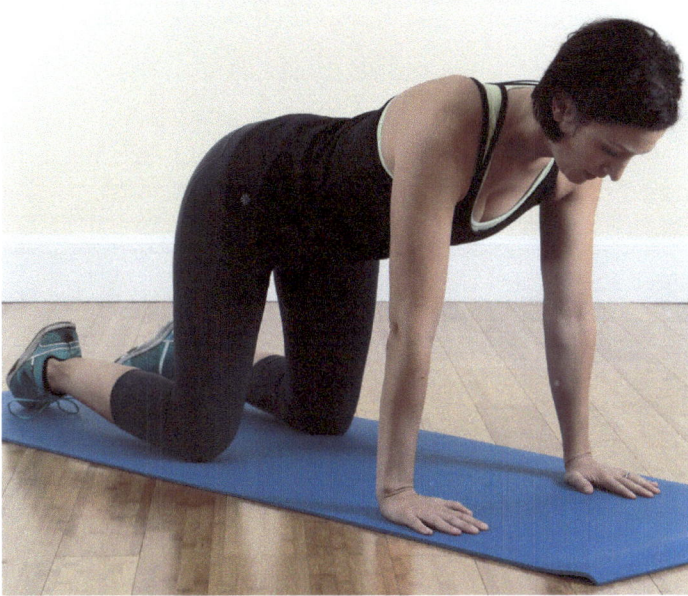

3A.
PreTrain Bird Dog. Start with a quadruped position. Perform a PreTrain Brace and PreTrain Shoulder Brace.

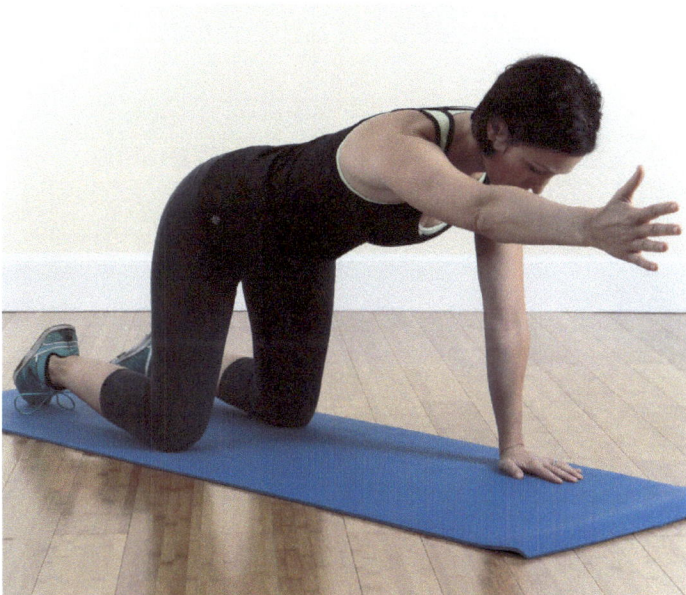

3B.
Keeping shoulders and PreTrain Brace engaged, use the muscles in your back to "pull" your arm forward. Feel the muscles in your shoulders work to lift your arm up, not going past your ear.

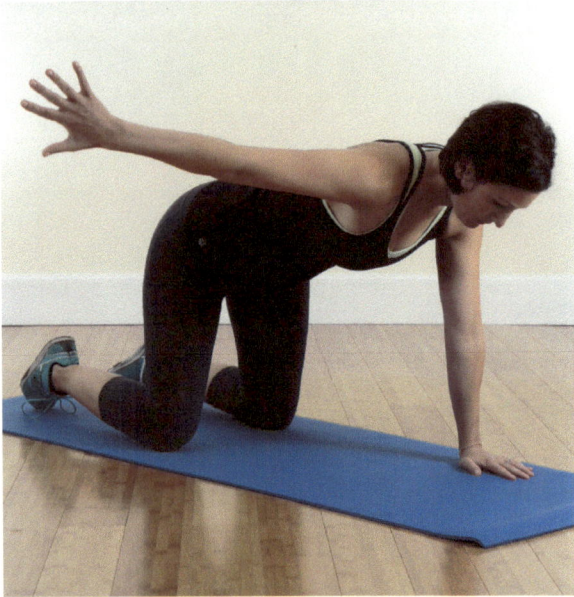

3C.
Keeping shoulders and the PreTrain Brace engaged, lift the arm out to the side. Keep your neck neutral and maintain stability throughout the core and back.

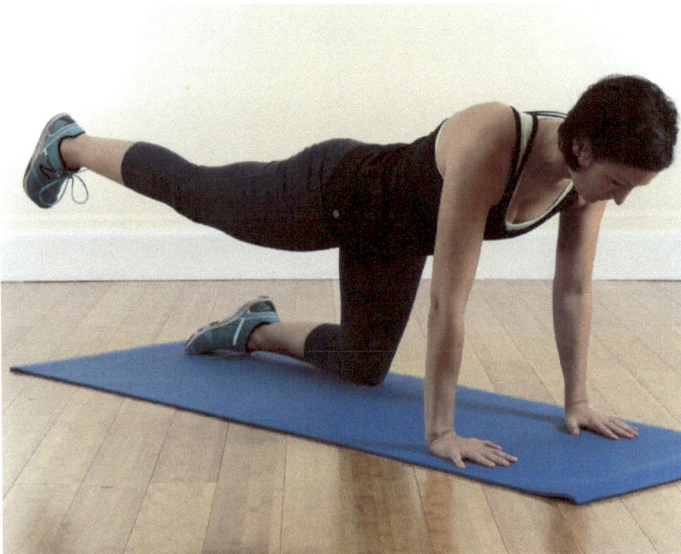

3D.
Make sure to keep your hips neutral, without arching your low back. Think about squeezing your glute to lift your leg.

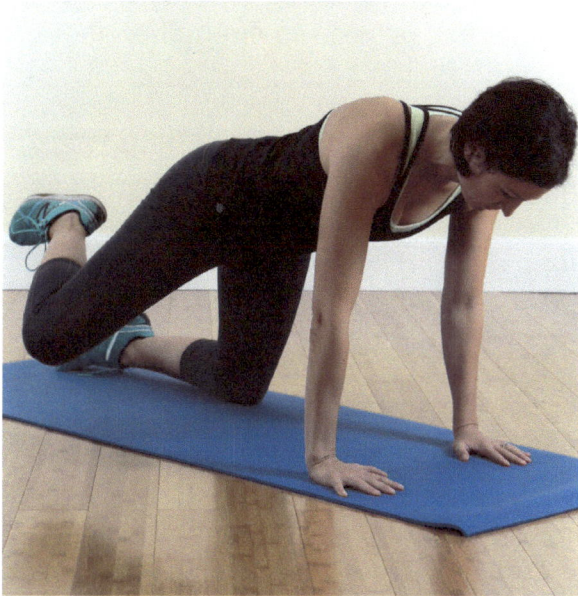

3E.
Maintaining PreTrain Brace and Shoulder Brace, squeeze your hip to lift your leg to the side. Do not lift past 30 degrees, and make sure to keep your low back straight and stable.

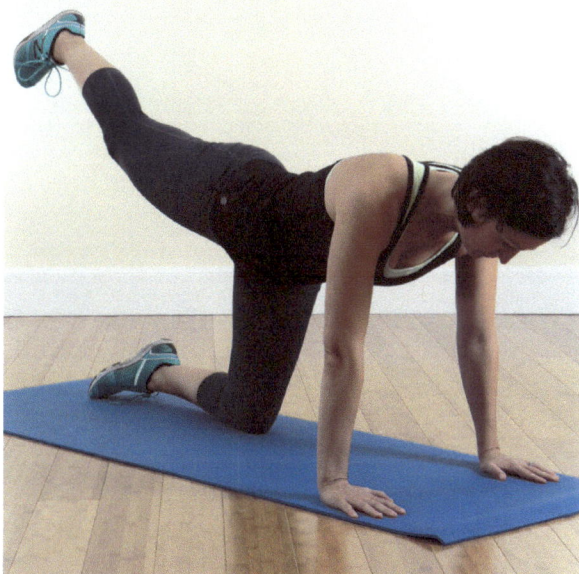

3F.
Common mistake. A common mistake is compromising core stability by lifting the leg too high. Your leg should stay in line with your hip and low back.

4. PreTrain Plank

A. Intention: This exercise is a modification of the traditional plank. The goal with this exercise is to build endurance in the stabilizing muscles of your hips, low back, and shoulder. By holding this exercise for a prolonged period of time, you are training these muscles not only to work, but to work for a longer period of time. Often with exercise, the stabilizing muscles aren't strong enough to stay working throughout a long workout. The PreTrain Plank is designed to strengthen these muscles for this purpose.

B. Description: Start in a quadruped position, but with your knees together. Walk your hands out in front of you so that your hands are still in line with your shoulders but your   knees are at a 45 degrees angle with the floor. Perform PreTrain Brace and Shoulder Brace. Squeeze your ankles and knees together to activate the groin muscles and your glute max. Make sure your low back stays in a neutral position, so that you are not arching or flattening your back. Hold strong for 30 seconds.

C. Common mistake: The importance here is perfect form. If you can only hold the plank for 5 seconds, then that is where you start. Build up to 30 seconds. Focus on recruiting all the major muscle groups in your hips, low back, shoulders, and core. If you begin to feel your hips sag and feel some stress in your low back, take a deep breath in and reset your PreTrain Brace. Really focus on squeezing the shoulder blades back and down together along with tightening the glute max and groin muscles on the inside of your thigh. Stay strong and breathe! If you continue to feel your hips sag, release the position, take note of the time you were able to stay in the position, and work to improve each time.

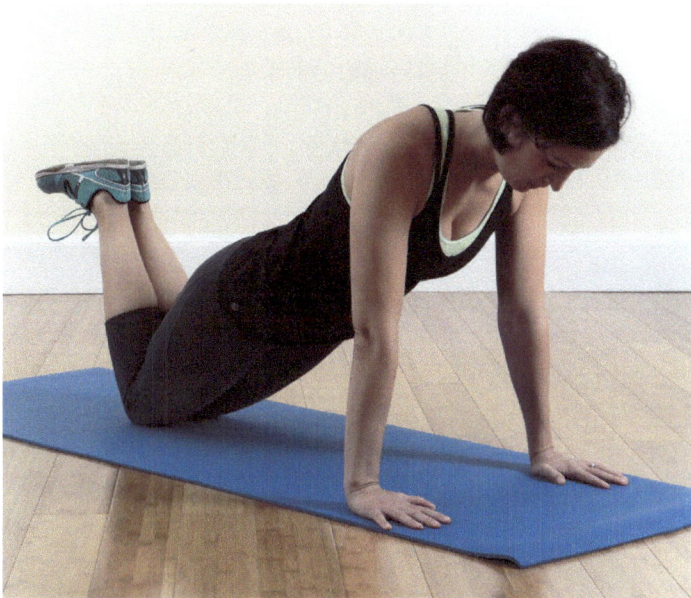

4A.
PreTrain Plank. Squeeze feet, knees, and hips together. Maintain a PreTrain Brace and Shoulder Brace. Keep neck neutral.

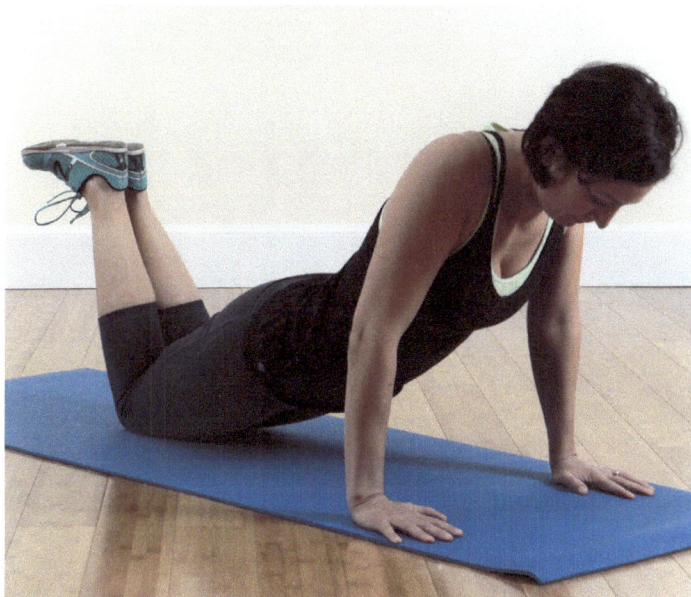

4B.
The most common mistake in performing the PreTrain Plank is to lose stability through the hips, core, and shoulders. If this happens, you will see your hips sag.

Module 1.2:

Bridging

A. Intention: This exercise is intended to begin stabilizing your pelvis and low back across your body, as with walking by alternating your leg movements. It works to improve your core stability while strengthening the glute max.

B. Description: Begin in the Level 1 bridging position. Activate the PreTrain Brace and lift your hips up into a bridge, squeezing the glute max and breathing out as you lift. When your hips are at a 45 degree angle, slowly straighten your right leg. Make sure to keep your pelvis stable and your hips level as you raise your right leg. Do not allow your right hip to dip down toward the floor as your straighten your right leg. Consciously contract the PreTrain Brace to stabilize the pelvis to prevent this. In a controlled manner, bend the right knee and bring the hips back down to a hook-lying position. Repeat with the left leg. Repeat for 10 repetitions.

C. Common mistakes: This is a very challenging exercise, especially with people who have a history of low back pain. However, it can also be one of the most effective exercises, and if you can master it, you will have a notable improvement with your stability and strength in your low back. The key to this exercise is to keep the hips stable and level, parallel to the floor. If you are having difficulty with this piece, you may modify the exercise by pressing the opposite foot of the leg you are moving, into the floor to contract the glute max. For example, if you are straightening the right leg, you may press the left foot, feeling the left glute tighten to "help" stabilize the pelvis. As with Level 1, if you feel any tightness or cramping in the hamstring, move the heel of your foot closer to your buttock.

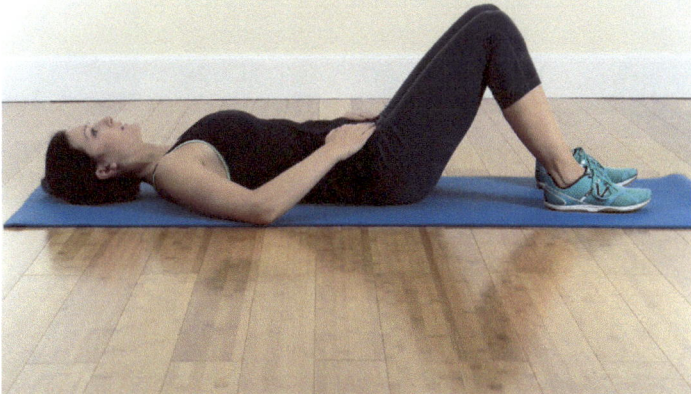

1A.
Lay on your back in a hook-lying position. Perform a PreTrain Brace.

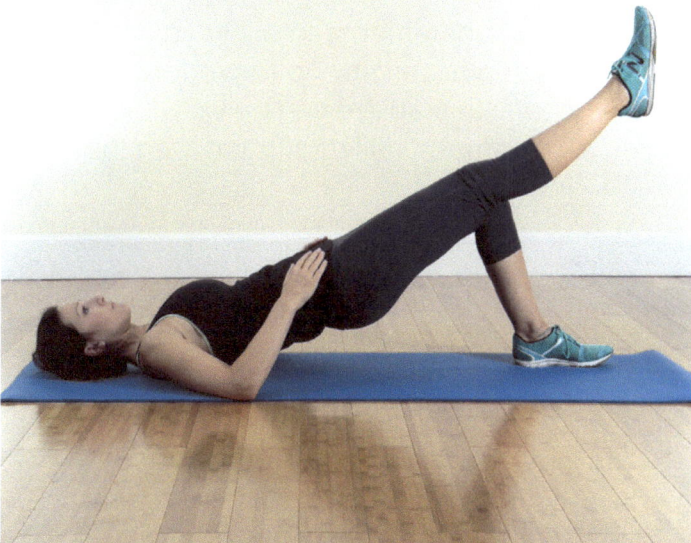

1B.
Lift your hips off the floor to a 45 degree angle. At the top of the 45 degree angle, straighten your right leg. Make sure to keep your PreTrain Brace strong and make sure your hips stay stable.

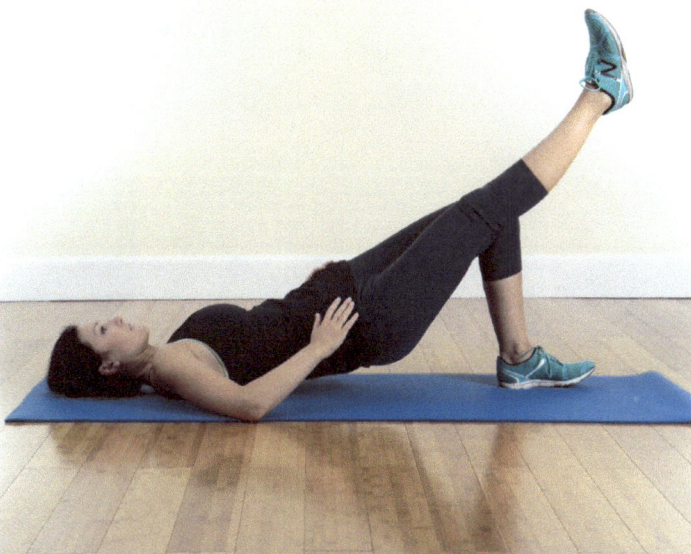

1C.
Common mistake. A common mistake is not maintaining a strong PreTrain Brace throughout the exercise, which will result in your hip dipping down towards the floor.

2. Dead Bug

A. Intention: This exercise begins to train your core, utilizing the PreTrain Brace, to be stable with movements that mimic every day walking and running. It begins to train "cross-body" stability that requires one side of your body to be stable while your opposite side moves.

B. Description: Begin with lying in a hook-lying position. Place palms of hands on the front of your hip bones. This will serve as a guide. Perform a PreTrain Brace. Maintaining the PreTrain Brace, lift one foot off the floor no more than 6 inches with a count of two seconds, and lower with a count of three seconds. The PreTrain Brace should hold your pelvis stable and your hips should not move. Alternate legs. Movements should be slow and steady. Perform 10 each side.

C. Common mistakes: Make sure your hips stay stable throughout the exercise, and that they do not move with leg movement. If you are having a hard time keeping your hips stable, as a temporary modification, you can press the opposite foot from the leg you are moving into the floor to recruit the glute max to help stabilize your pelvis. For example, if you are lifting your right foot, you can press your whole left foot into the floor to help. Be careful not to allow your left hip to rise off the floor. This is just a temporary modification. To move forward throughout the program, however, you must be able to stabilize you pelvis without this "help." Take your time with this exercise. It can be challenging for even the best conditioned athletes.

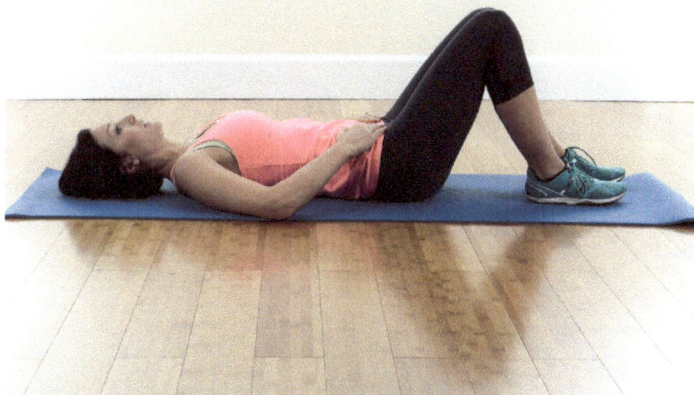

2A.
Start lying in a hook-lying position. Perform a PreTrain Brace.

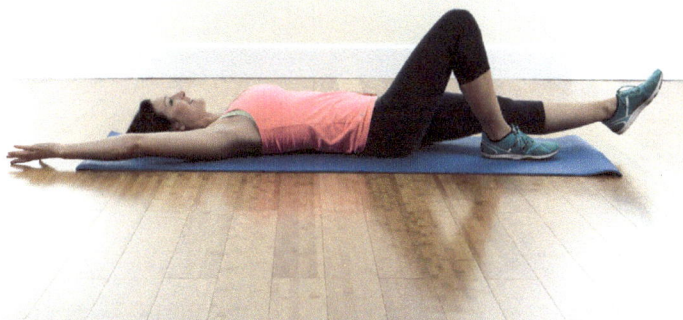

2B.
Keeping your PreTrain Brace engaged, slowly lift your foot off the floor. Keep your hands on your hip bones to serve as a guide. Your hands, and your hips, should stay stable.

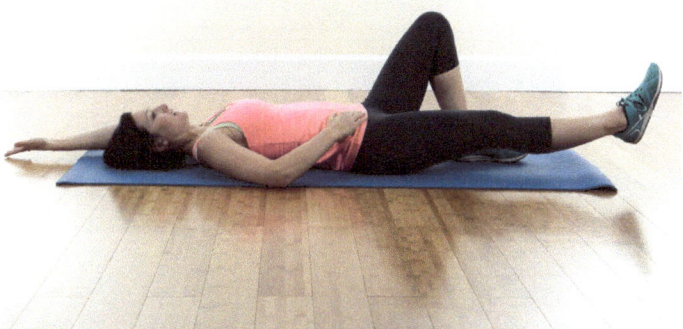

2C.
Common mistake: A common mistake is to not properly stabilize your core with the PreTrain Brace. You will see the right hip dip towards the floor as you life your right leg if your core is not properly engaged.

3. PreTrain Bird Dog

A. Intention: The exercise builds on the challenge of stabilizing the shoulder and core while adding in the challenge of gravity. This exercise really coordinates the major stabilizing muscles throughout your low back and shoulders to move in a strong, stable manner.

B. Description: Bird Dog Level 2 is similar to Bird Dog Level 1. Begin in the quadruped position with knees under hips and hands slightly wider than shoulder width. Perform the PreTrain Brace and Shoulder Brace. Slide your right leg back behind you, squeezing the glute max to lift the leg. Simultaneously, bring your left arm straight above your head so your elbow is near your ear, with your thumb pointed up to the ceiling. Maintain stability. Return to the quadruped position slowly, controlling your motion. Tap the floor with your right knee and your left hand. Keeping the right knee bent, lift the knee out to the side no more than 30 degrees, contracting the deep hip muscles. Simultaneously, bring your left arm out to the side, with thumb pointed to the floor, and squeeze your left shoulder blade in towards your spine. Return to the quadruped position.

Repeat with right leg/left arm combination and alternate with left leg/right arm. Repeat 5 times.

C. Common mistakes: Level 2 builds on the coordination patterns established in Level 1. In Level 2, we focus on stabilizing the shoulders with the pelvis and low back while strengthening the bigger muscles in these areas at the same time. Make sure your back stays parallel to the floor throughout the movements. If you need to, modify the exercise by only moving the arms and legs as high as you can without compromising the straight back.

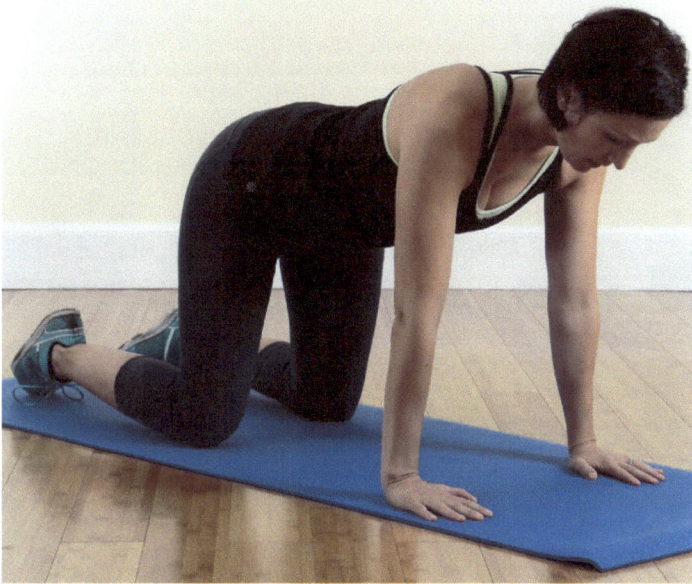

3A.
Start in the quadruped position. Perform a PreTrain Brace and Shoulder Brace to engage the core and shoulder stabilizing muscles together.

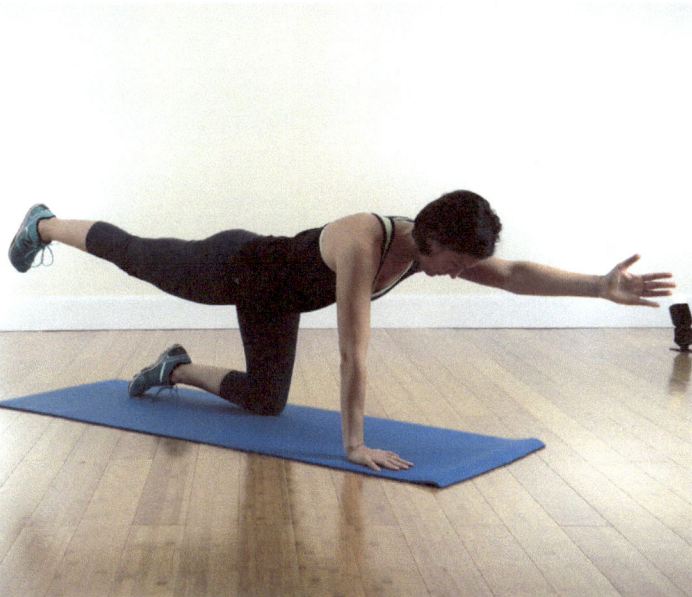

3B.
Maintaining contraction of the PreTrain Brace and Shoulder Brace, raise your arm in front of you, no higher than ear level. At the same time, contract your opposite glute and lift your leg behind you. Return to the quadruped position (on your hands and knees).

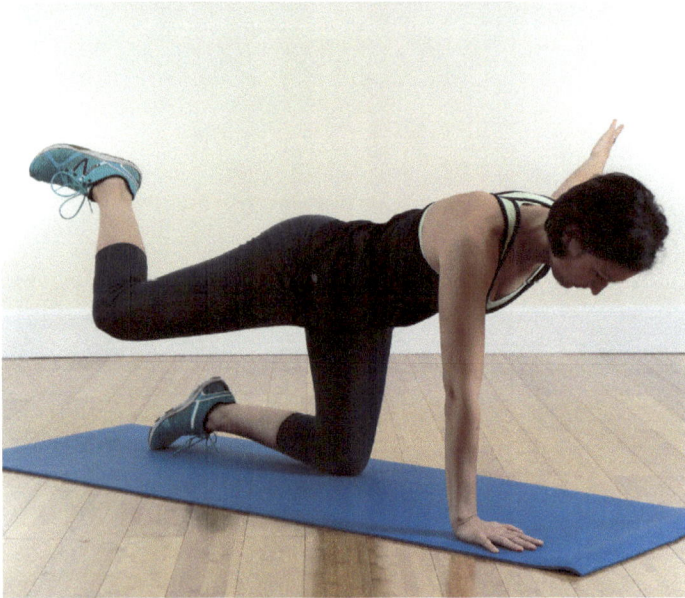

3C.
Continue with the PreTrain Brace and Shoulder Brace. Lift your arm out to the side, using your shoulder muscles to pull your arm up to about ear level. Keeping your opposite knee bent, lift your knee to the side, squeezing your hip muscles. Do not lift past 30 degrees.

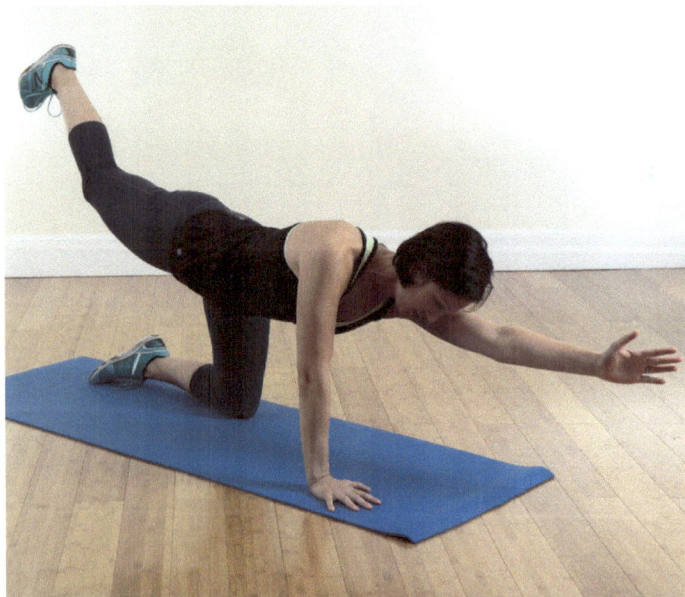

3D.
Common mistake. Common mistakes include lifting the leg too high, which indicates there is a loss of stability in the core and hips.

4. PreTrain Push Up

A. Intention: This exercise strengthens the whole upper back while maintaining stability throughout the back and hips.

B. Description: Begin in the PreTrain Plank position, with PreTrain Brace and Shoulder Brace engaged. Slowly lower your upper body down to the floor and lower your feet to the floor at the same time, controlling each motion. As you push up, also contract the glute max, bending the knees to return to the starting position. Make sure your low back stays strong and neutral. Do not arch, or hyperextend, your back when you press up. Focus on the muscles in your mid back, in between your shoulder blades, "pulling" you up rather than on the muscles in the front of your chest "pushing" you up. Move slowly and with intention. Repeat 10 times.

C. Common mistakes: Make sure to keep the neck neutral and don't strain your neck.   To modify, only do as many push ups as you can until you can build up to 10 repetitions. Focus on doing one more push up each time you perform the program. Keep your back straight and don't let your hips dip.

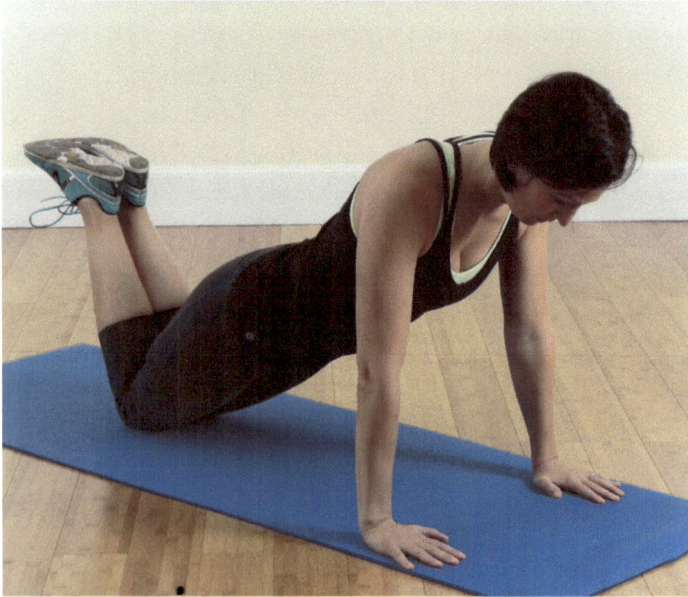

4A.
In a modified push up position, squeeze your feet and knees together. Perform a PreTrain Brace and Shoulder Brace in the push up position.

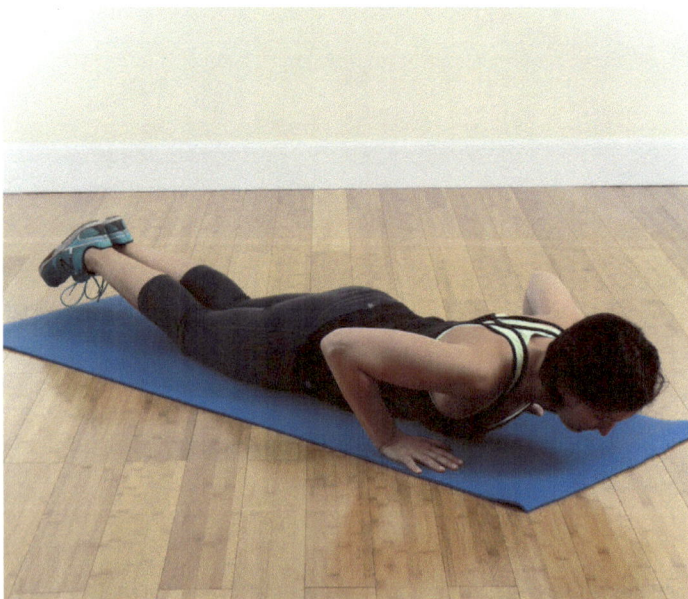

4B
Lower your upper body to the floor and, at the same time, lower your legs to the floor.

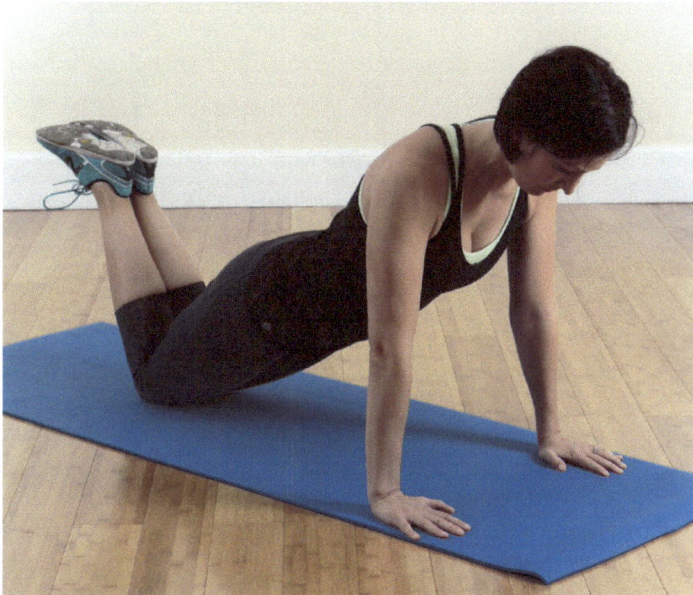

4C.
As you push up from the floor, squeeze your glutes, while simultaneously pressing your feet and knees together.

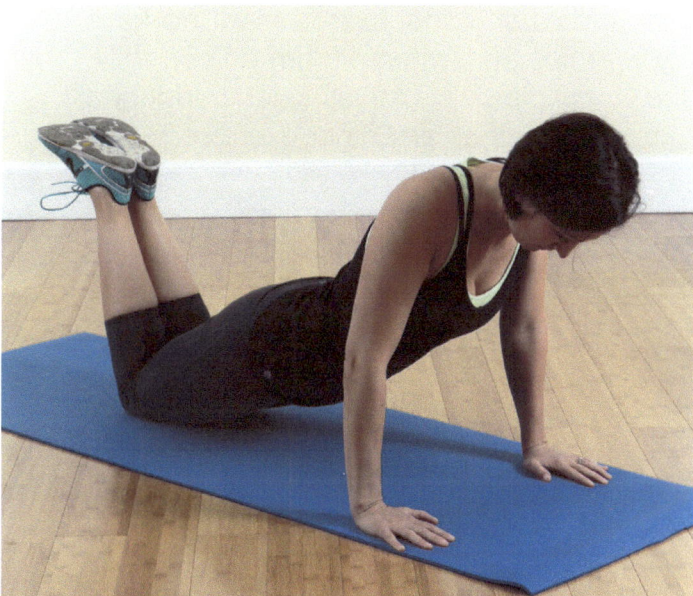

4D.
Common mistake. Don't let your hips sag, or let your low back arch. Keep your pelvis and low back neutral.

Congratulations! You've successfully made it through *Module 1: Rebuild*. You now have the foundation of stability within the shoulders and core. Time to apply these new techniques and improved strength to *Module 2: Restore*. Keep movin' forward!

"Learning proper movement is like hitting the 'reset' button on your body."

This series of exercises will help you undo compensations and restore correct movement patterns.

Module 2: Restore has two levels of progression. Each level has a set of four exercises that should be performed successively. Each set should be repeated three times at least four times per week. *Module 2.1.1: Flexibility and Mobility* that accompanies Module 2 can be performed either on the "off days" of the workouts, or on the same day.

1. Reverse squat series
A. Intention: The squat is one of the most utilized exercises in fitness. However, most people perform it incorrectly. It isn't necessarily their fault. Well-meaning instructors may modify a client's position by elevating their heels or pulling their hips back to promote hip flexibility. You should be able to perform a squat without modifications. If you find yourself needing to use alternatives such as those listed above, it is an indication there is an issue with your flexibility, stability, or strength. That is why this module includes a flexibility component. As we increase the number of muscle groups working, we need to make sure there is flexibility in the right areas.

The squat is the only exercise that targets the entire posterior chain, which are all the muscles in the back of your legs, hips, and back. Other exercises will address these muscles, but the squat is the only exercise that, when performed correctly, will completely work the entire sequence of muscles. The squat, when performed correctly, will protect and support the knees more than any other exercise.[3]

To teach the squat, we begin with movements everyone can perform and guide you into the correct form. There are acceptable modifications, which we will mention, on your path to the perfect squat. This exercise requires flexibility throughout the hips, lower extremity, and mid back, stability in the core and shoulders, and strength in the hips and lower extremity.

B. Description: Begin by standing with feet 1 and 1/2 shoulder width apart with feet pointed straight forward, arms to the side. "Lock in" the stability with your feet and ankles using the Lower Extremity Brace. Bend down at the waist, keeping your knees slightly bent, and touch your hands to the floor. Drop your buttocks down until you are into a squat, making sure your knees are in line or behind your knees. Raise your arms in front of you, locking in your shoulders with the Shoulder Brace. Keep your low back straight, and make sure your weight is dispersed evenly throughout both feet. Perform a PreTrain Brace and exhale as you contract your glutes, quads, and hamstrings to push yourself up into a standing position. Repeat 10 times.

C. Common mistakes: Only squat down as far as you can without bending at the back. The ultimate goal is to get your thighs below your knees, while keeping your knees behind your toes. However, if you can't get your thighs below your knees, work to get your thighs parallel to the floor. Keep your back straight, your core engaged, and your shoulders strong. A proper deep squat requires flexibility in all the major muscles, and mobility in the feet, ankle and hips. It also requires strong core and glute coordination. This exercise is building on the previous exercises in that it requires this coordination with the additional challenge of weight bearing stability.

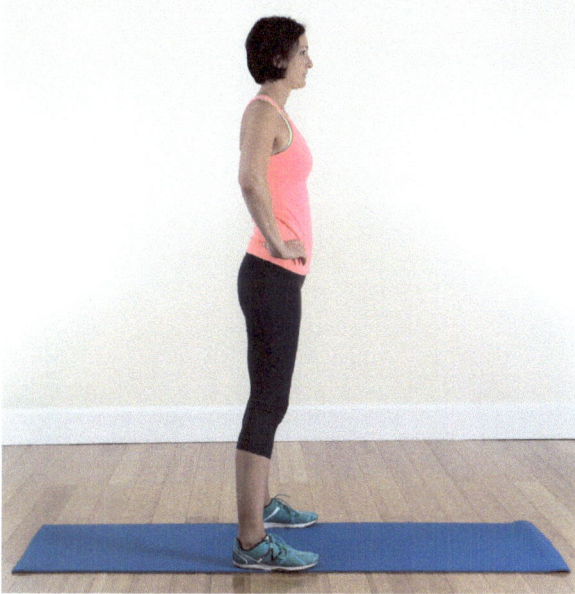

1A.
Start standing, engaging your PreTrain Brace, and Lower Extremity Brace.

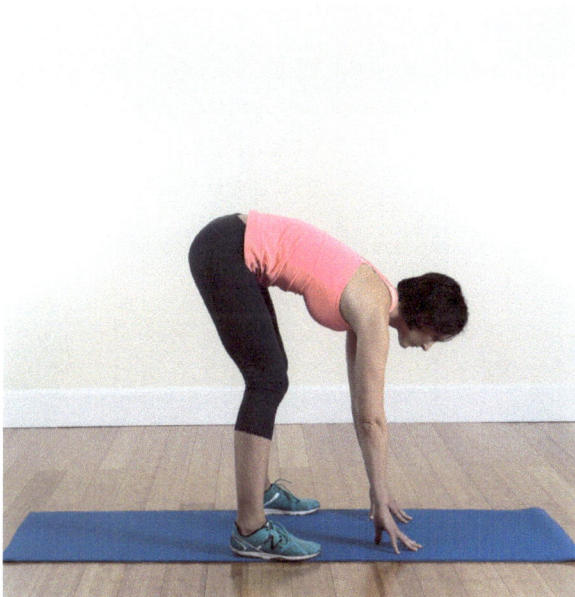

1B.
Keeping your knees slightly bent, bend forward at your waist to touch the floor.

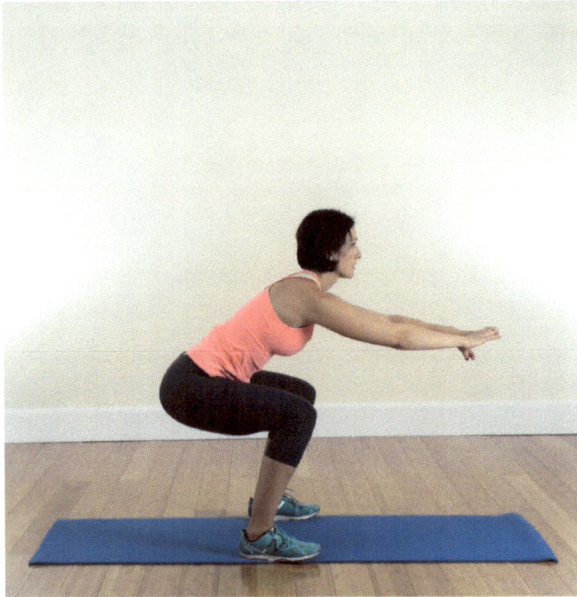

1C.
Slowly, lower your hips down to a squatting position, and lift your arms in front of you.

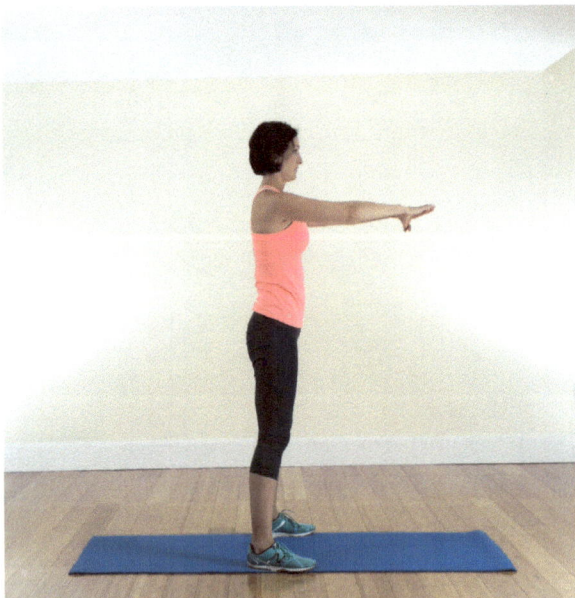

1D.
Breathing out, press your feet into the floor, and squeeze your glutes to move into a standing position. Make sure to keep your shoulders engaged.

2. Reverse lunge series, single lunge

A. Intention: This exercise begins to incorporate balance with strength and mobility. By moving each leg backwards, you are requiring the core and glute complex to respond to a one-legged stance. By keeping both glutes engaged throughout the exercise, you are able to enhance the stretch in the front of the thigh with the back leg, and strengthen the glute in the front leg. Core stability and cross body stability with hip and back strength is emphasized.

B. Description: Begin standing with feet shoulder width apart. Perform a PreTrain Brace. Keeping your hands on your hips, perform a Shoulder Brace to keep your upper back muscles engaged. Bring your right leg back behind you, bending the knee to touch the floor. The front leg will also bend and make sure to keep the knee behind your toe. Focus on contracting both the front and back glute as you press up, noting the stretch in the front of the hip in your back leg. Press up and bring the back leg up to the front to a standing position, making sure to keep the PreTrain Brace to improve balance. Repeat with the opposite leg going back. Repeat 10 times.

C. Common mistakes: Go slow with this exercise. Try to get your knee down to the floor. However, if you are having difficulty with this, get the knee as far to the floor as possible and be mindful of improving your flexibility. Watch to make sure your front knee doesn't go in front of the toes.

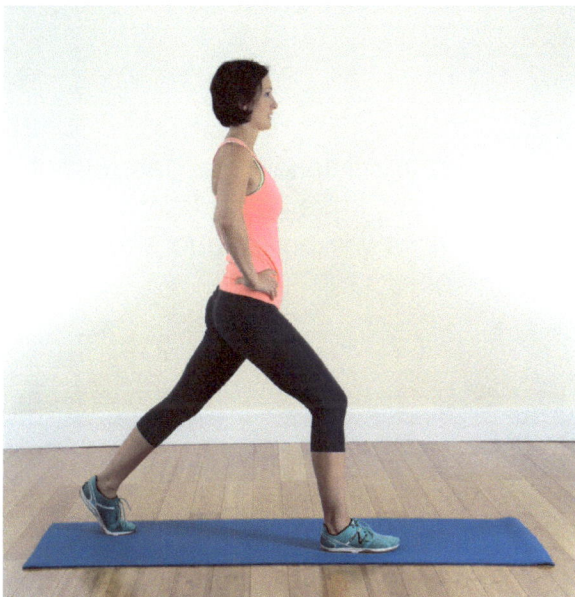

2A.
Bring one leg back behind you, keeping your PreTrain and Shoulder Brace engaged.

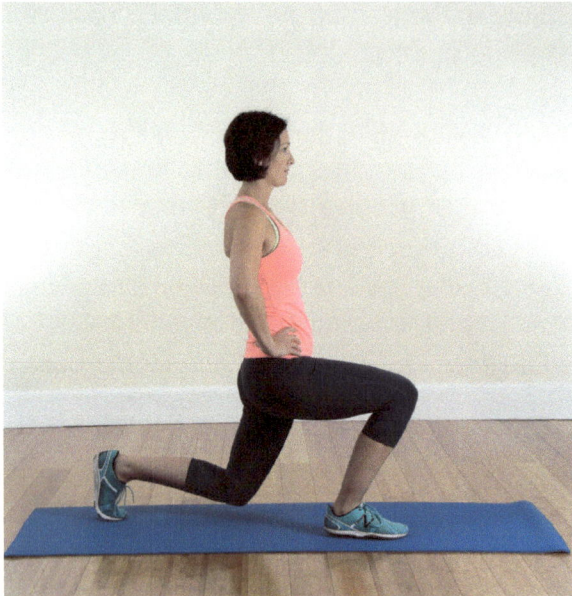

2B.
Bend the back knee, trying to get it as close to the ground as possible. Do not let your front knee go past your front toe. Press up back into a standing position, squeezing your glutes and breathing out as you press up.

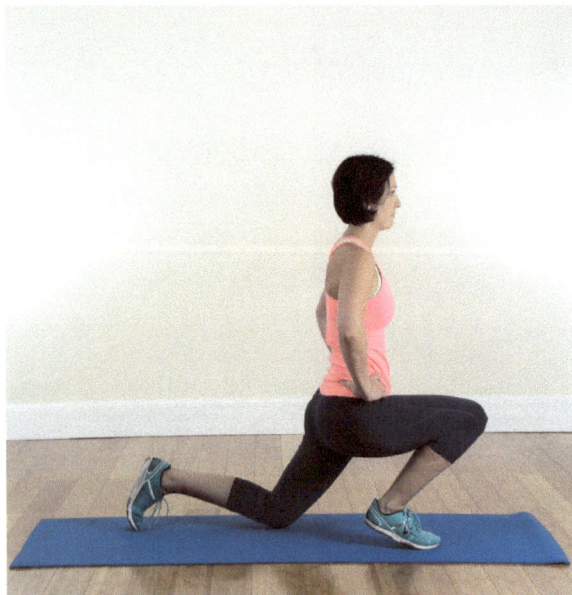

2C.
Common mistake. Be careful not to let your knee go in front of your toe. This will put undue stress on the knee.

3. Deadlift series

A. Intention: The deadlift is a fantastic exercise. It strengthens the posterior chain, which includes all the major muscles in your back and lower legs. It works almost every muscle from the foot through the back and into the shoulders. It requires flexibility in the hips and ankles, and a very strong and stable core.

B. Description: Stand with your feet pointing forward and about shoulder width apart. "Lock in" your stability with a Lower Extremity Brace. Put your right hand behind your lower back and your left hand over your left shoulder attempting to touch your right hand. This will serve as a guide to make sure your low back stays straight and strong. Bend your torso forward at your waist and bend your knees slightly, keeping your neck neutral. Shift your weight slightly toward your heels as you bend forward. Perform a PreTrain Brace and exhale as you push your hip forward, driving your heels into the ground, and lifting your torso upright without moving your spine, straightening your legs at the same time. Move slowly and tighten your glutes as you lift your torso up. You will do this for the first round of three sets. Repeat 10 times.

C. Common mistakes: The dead lift can be intimidating. However, this is an exercise everyone can learn how to do, and this will strengthen the low back and hips considerably. Go slowly and work on getting perfect form, hinging the hips so they float behind you while keeping your back straight. You will most likely be a little sore in your hamstring and hips the following day! Along with core, hip, and mid back stability, this exercise will engage the small but very important multifidi muscles in the low back. These muscles are very important in holding the spine stable at each vertebra. This exercise needs to be performed slowly to keep these muscles engaged.

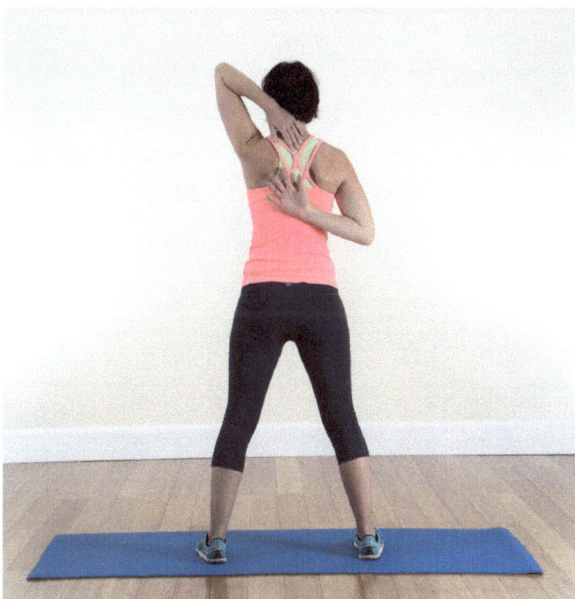

3A.
Start by intertwining your hands behind your back, with one arm going above your shoulder, and the other going behind your low back. Perform a PreTrain Brace and Lower Extremity Brace to activate the core and legs.

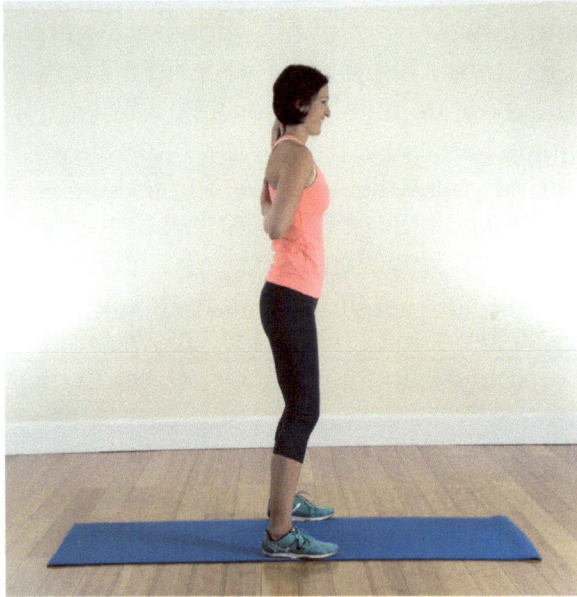

3A.1
Start by intertwining your hands behind your back, with one arm going above your shoulder, and the other going behind your low back. Perform a PreTrain Brace and Lower Extremity Brace to activate the core and legs.

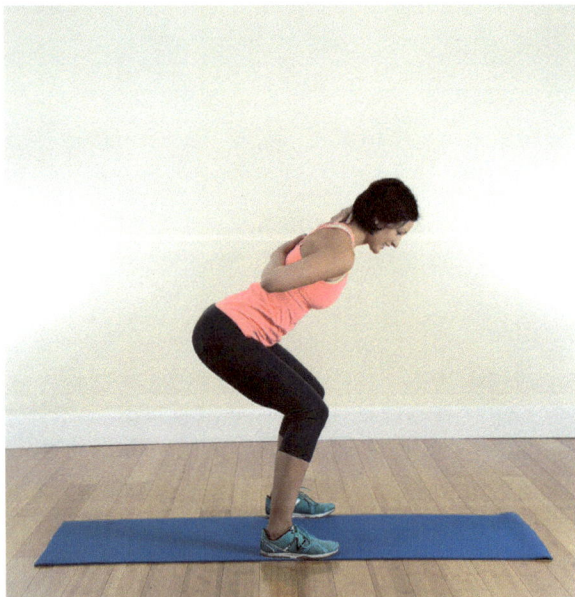

3B.
Keeping your back straight, bend your knees and move your hips back. Your hands will serve as a guide to make sure your back stays straight.

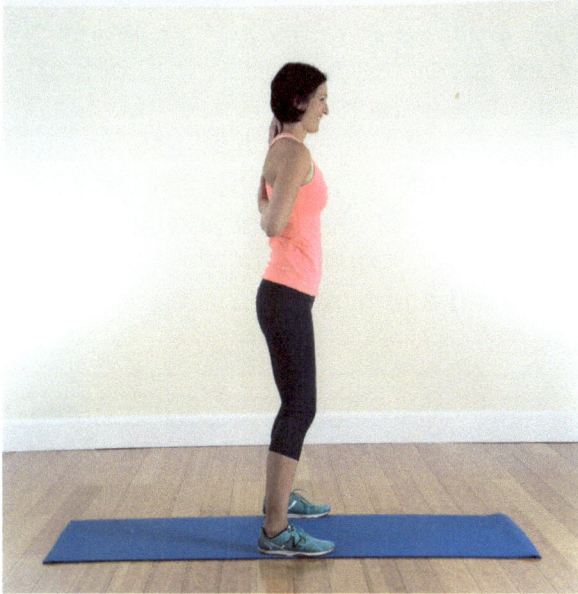

3C.
Press your feet into the floor, breathing out while you press up through your legs into a standing position. Keep your core muscles engaged.

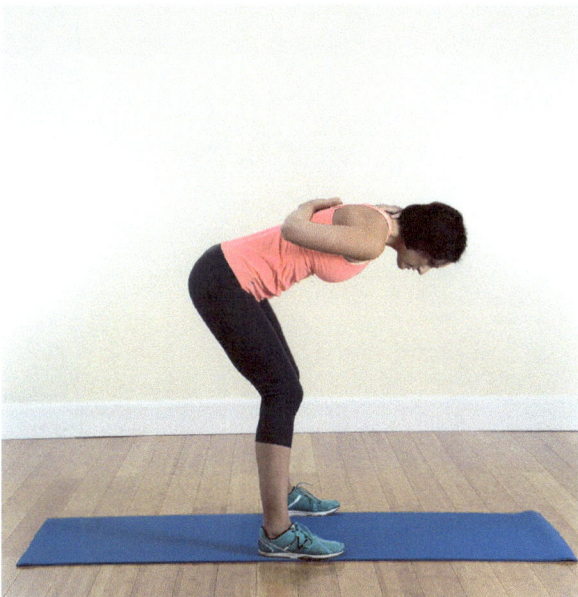

3D.
Common mistake. The most common mistake is moving through your low back rather than your hips. Focus on moving your hips back behind you as you bend your knees, rather than focusing on just bending down.

4. Windmills

A. Intention: The Windmill is a common exercise with Kettlebell workouts. It is a challenging exercise in that it requires hip mobility, shoulder and core stability, and shoulder mobility. It challenges shoulder and core stability in different planes of movement to train your body to be stable in many different directions.

B. Description: Stand with your feet double width apart with your toes pointing forward. Turn your left foot 45 degrees so it is pointed to your left. "Lock in" the stability with your foot and ankle with the Lower Extremity Brace. Maintain PreTrain Brace and Shoulder Brace, raising your right hand with a straight arm to the ceiling, turning your head to maintain eye contact on this hand. Hinge your left hip back, bending your front knee. Keeping your left leg bent and your right leg straight, drop your left hand to the ground as your continue raising your right to the ceiling. Touch the floor with your left hand and slowly, drive back to the starting position. Repeat 10 times each side.

C. Common mistakes: Don't collapse your torso. Make sure your core is strong and stable throughout the movement. To modify, go as close to the floor as possible. If you have a difficult time reaching the floor with your hand, it is an indication that you will need to spend more time with the flexibility/mobility module.

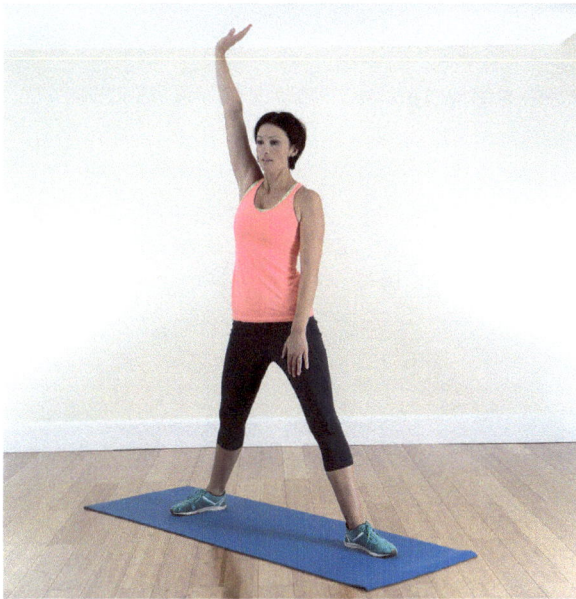

4A.
Stand with a neutral spine, engaging the PreTrain Brace and Lower Extremity Brace.

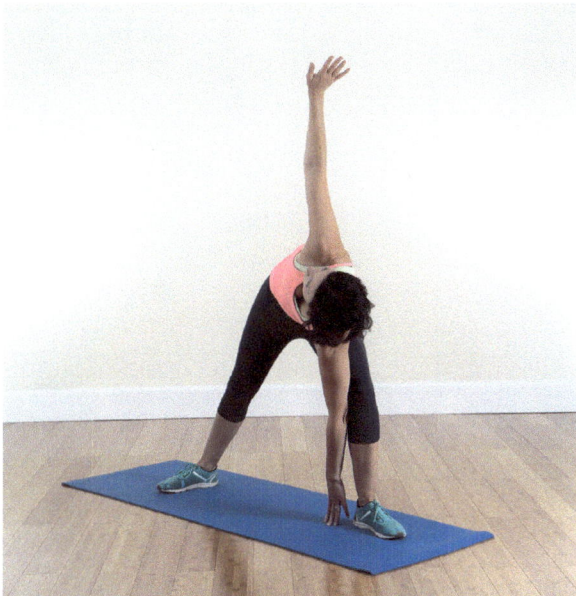

4B.
Bend your front knee and lower your left hand to the floor. Bring your opposite hand above you, and turn your head to look at the ceiling.

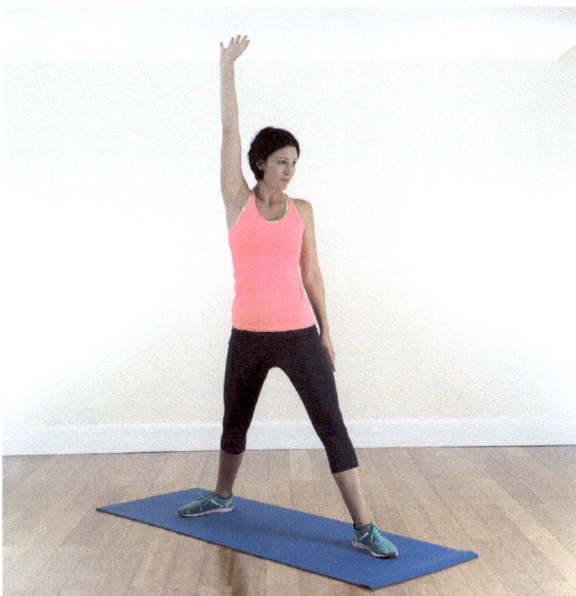

4C.
Press up with both feet, turn your body, keeping your core engaged and breathing out. Think about extending up to the ceiling and staying long and stable. Then, turn to look over your left toe.

Module 2.2

1. Reverse squat series - reverse squat with press up

A. Intention: Good things are worth mastering, and the squat is one of them. In this level, we have included an arm movement to challenge your shoulders as well as your lower extremity strength, stability, and flexibility.

B. Description: Begin by standing with feet 1 and 1/2 shoulder width apart with feet pointed straight forward, arms to the side. "Lock in" with your feet and ankles using the Lower Extremity Brace. Bend down at the waist. Keeping your knees straight and while touching your hands to the floor, drop your buttocks down to a squat form. Make sure your knees are in line with your toes. This time, rotate your arms so that the palms of your hands are facing the ceiling and are at the level of your ears. Brace your shoulders, with the Shoulder Brace to activate the stabilizing muscles of the shoulder. Keep your low back straight, and make sure your weight is dispersed evenly throughout your feet. Perform a PreTrain Brace and exhale as you use contract your glutes, quads, and hamstrings to push yourself up into a standing position. As you move to a standing position, press up to the ceiling with your hands, straightening your arms overhead. Repeat 10 times.

C. Common mistakes: Make sure to keep your knees behind toes and your back straight as your hips go back and rotate. To modify, go as far down as you can, trying to improve on each repetition.

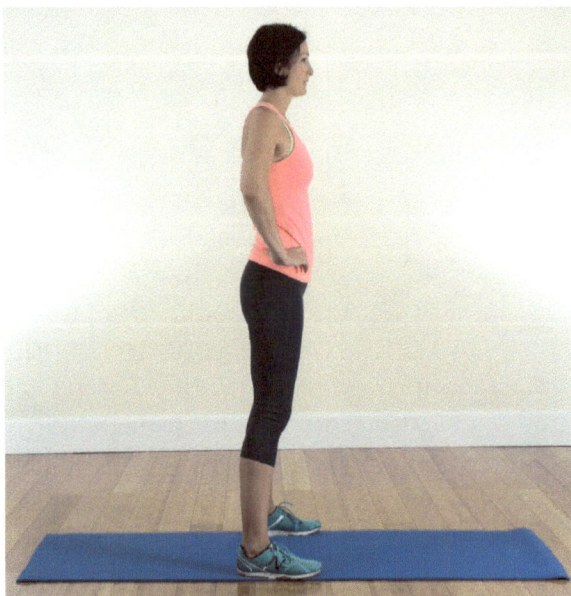

1A.
Start standing, engaging your PreTrain Brace, and Lower Extremity Brace.

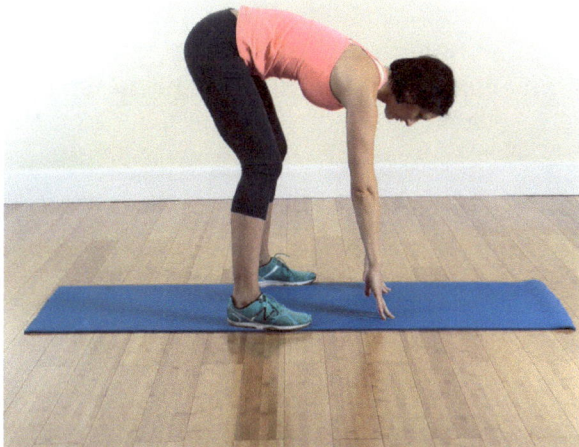

1B.
Keeping your knees slightly bent, bend forward at your waist to touch the floor.

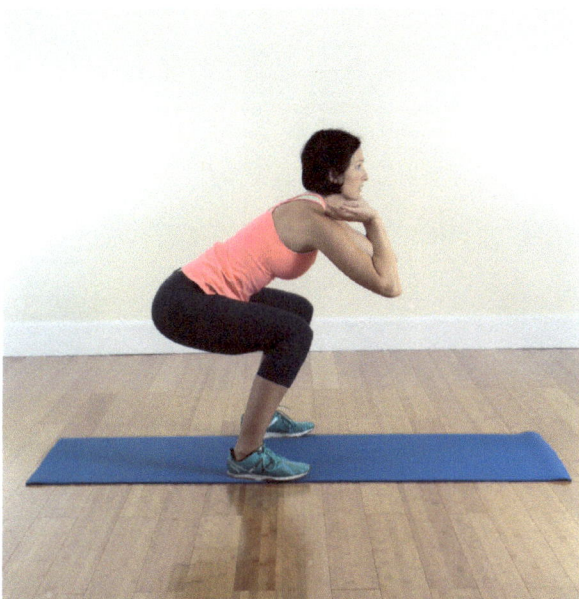

1C.
Shift your hips back behind you and move your hands by your ears. Your elbows will be pointing out in front of you.

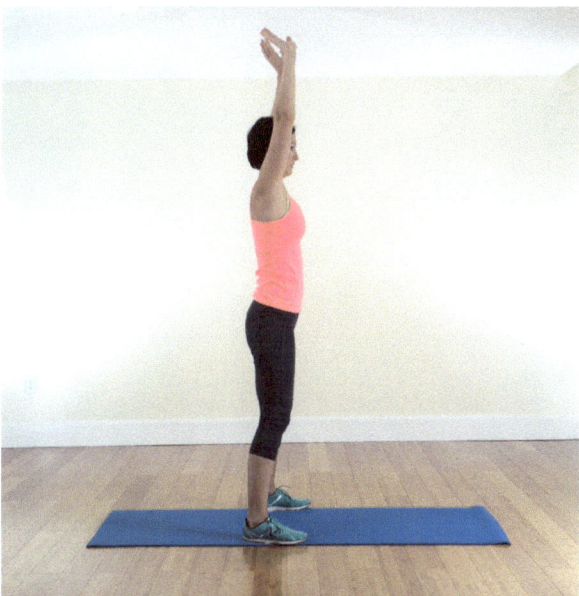

1D.
Focus on pressing your feet into the floor, squeezing your glutes, and press up to the ceiling as you stand. Breathe out as you move through the movement.

2. Reverse lunge series - with arm movement

A. Intention: By engaging the shoulder and mid back stabilizers, the arms will seem to "float" over your head. The muscles in your back are actually "lifting up" your arms. Your neck should be relaxed. This exercise strengthens your bigger muscle groups in your hips and low back while challenging cross body stability. This exercise improves full body balance and flexibility in the lower body while strengthening the core and upper body.

B. Description: Perform the PreTrain Brace with reverse lunge as described in level 1. As you step back, perform a Shoulder Brace as you raise both arms above your head. Lower the arms as you step back to a normal stance. Repeat with opposite legs. Repeat 10 times.

C. Common mistakes: Don't move too fast with this exercise. The full value of this exercise is experienced when it is performed slowly and controlled. Watch that the front knee doesn't cross in front of the toes. Make sure the Shoulder Brace is engaged.

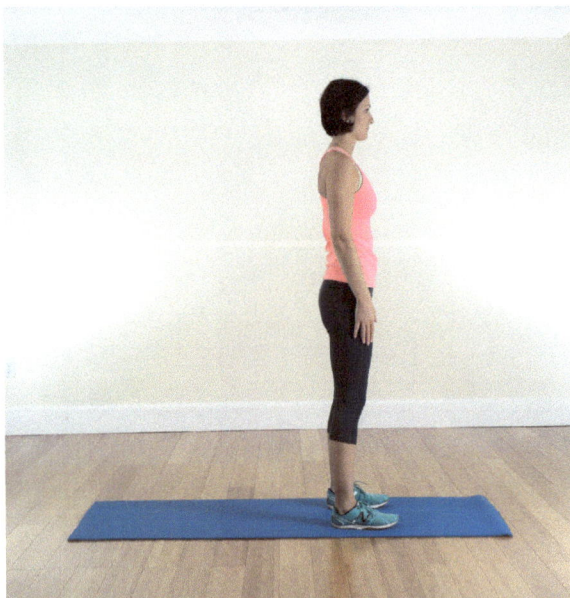

2A.
Start standing, and engage the PreTrain Brace.

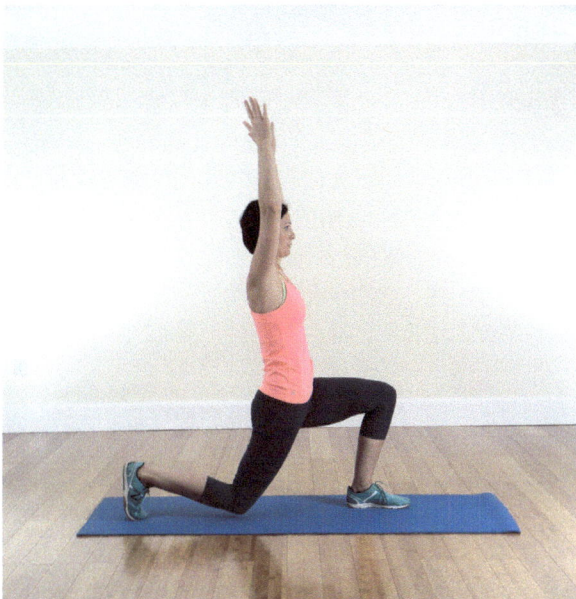

2B.
As you step back into a lunge, maintain the PreTrain Brace and lift your arms above your head. Feel your shoulders engage as you pull with your back muscles to lift your arms.

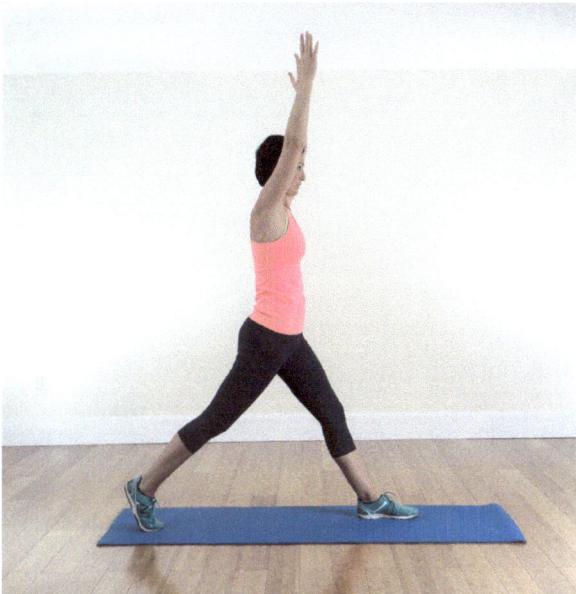

2C.
Press up through your legs and hips, breathing out as you press up. Feel your glutes contract to press up through the lunge. Alternate legs.

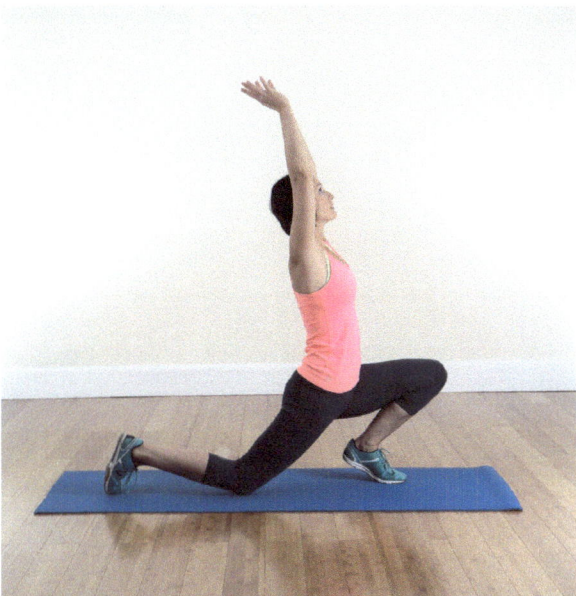

2D.
Common mistake. Common mistakes include overextending the low back and allowing the front knee to extend past the front toe.

3. Deadlift with row series - one-legged deadlift with row

This exercise requires the use of resistance bands.

A. Intention: The single-leg deadlift will add in the challenge of balance along with core and hip strength and stability. This exercise incorporates the bird dog exercise from Module 1, which requires stabilizing the pelvis and back by activating the core complex with the PreTrain Brace, and glute strength. In this exercise you will combine hip flexibility with balance training, posterior chain and core strengthening, and upper back strengthening.

B. Description: To begin, stand about shoulder width apart. Follow the instructions regarding anchoring the bands in a doorframe that were included in your band purchase. Make sure the door is shut properly and test the band before using. Perform the PreTrain Brace and Shoulder Brace, and "lock in" your foot and ankle stability with the Lower Extremity Brace. Keeping a medium tension on the bands, slowly lift your non-supporting leg behind you, keeping the core complex tight and your pelvis level. Make sure to keep your back straight, and lean forward from the hips, not the waist. Keep the front leg slightly bent and keep your knee "soft." Maintaining your Shoulder Brace, keep your arms in front of you until you feel a stretch in your hamstrings. Then, focus on driving your heel into the floor, maintaining the stability in your foot and ankle, and keep the core strong. As you slowly bring your back leg down, complete the movement by bending your elbows, bringing them back behind you into a row. Stay standing on one leg. Do 10 repetitions on one side. Repeat with opposite leg back.

C. Common mistakes: This exercise is best performed slowly with control. You will feel your low back muscles working. Use the skills learned in Module 1 to maintain PreTrain Brace and pelvic stability. Make sure your pelvis stays stable and does not twist to the right or left with the exercise. This is challenging but will improve balance and coordination.

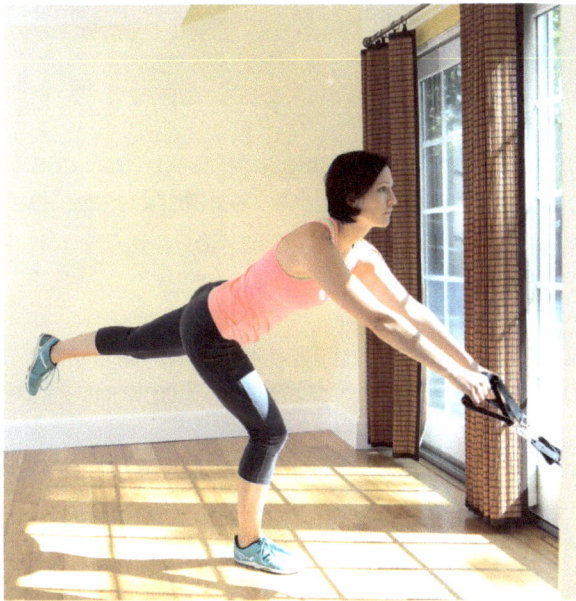

3A.
Maintain a strong stance by pressing your right foot into the floor and engaging your shoulders with a Shoulder Brace. Keeping your pelvis level and your core tight, raise your left leg back behind you by squeezing your glute.

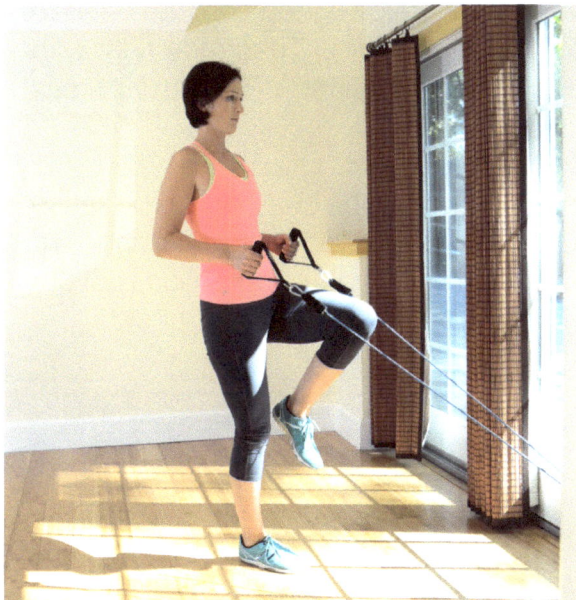

3B.
Slow and controlled, bring your back leg up into a high knee. Complete the movement by bending your elbows, bringing them back behind you into a row. Stay standing on one leg.

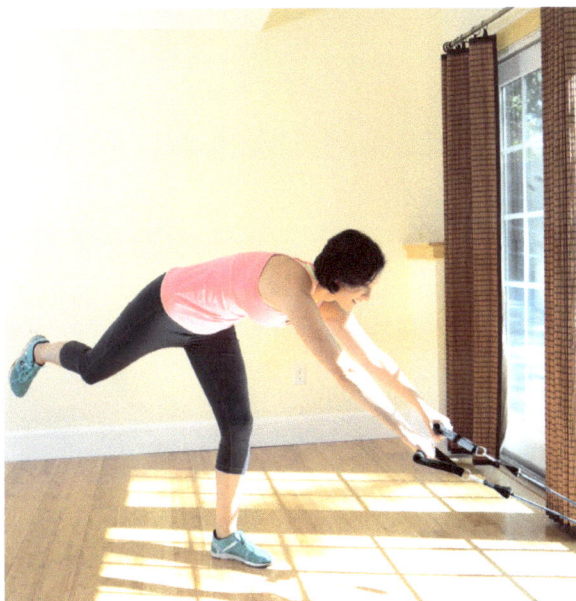

3C.
Common mistake. This is a challenging exercise. The most common mistake is to lose stability from the leg up through the core, and therefore lose form. Watch that you don't hunch over to grab the bands, and that you are engaging your glutes to lift your back leg.

4. Windmill series - resistance bands

This exercise requires the use of resistance bands.

A. Intention: This is a fantastic shoulder stabilizing exercise. It also requires flexibility in hips and stability in the core. The addition of the resistance band increases the challenge for shoulder stability. Be mindful to not engage the neck muscles with this exercise.

B. Description: Stand with your feet double width apart with your toes pointing forward. Turn your left foot 45 degrees so it is pointed to your left. "Lock in" the stability with your foot and ankle with the Lower Extremity Brace. Secure the resistance band by looping one handle through the other, so there is only one handle available to grab. Grab this handle with your left hand, while maintaining moderate tension on the band. Maintain PreTrain Brace and Shoulder Brace, raising your right hand with a straight arm to the ceiling, turning your head to maintain eye contact on this hand. Hinge your left hip back, bending your front knee. Keeping your left leg bent and your right leg straight, drop your left hand to the ground as you continue raising your right to the ceiling. Touch the floor with your left hand and slowly, drive back to the starting position. Repeat 10 times each side.

C. Common mistakes: Don't let your top hand move. It will be challenging because the band creates instability that require your shoulder muscles to respond. To keep it steady, engage your shoulders and make them stable. Turn to look at your top hand, keep neck relaxed. There shouldn't be any tension in your neck.

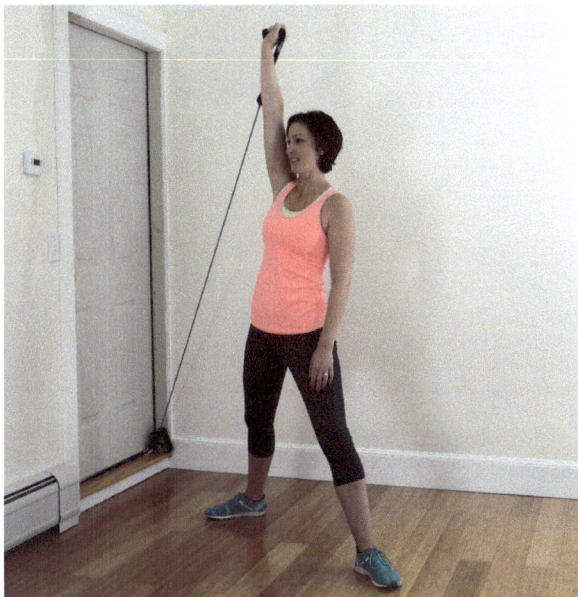

4A.
Begin with your left foot pointed out at a 90 degree angle. Lift your opposite arm above your head, maintaining tension on the band. Maintain a PreTrain Brace.

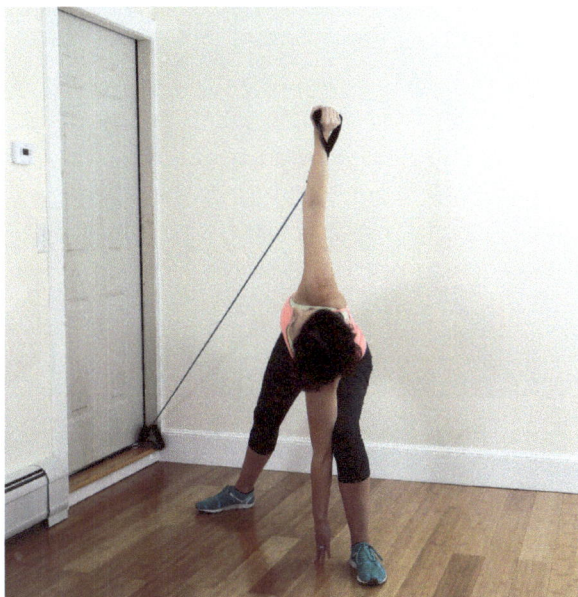

4B.
Keeping tension on your right hand and engaging your Shoulder Brace, bend the front knee and turn to look up at your top hand. Touch the floor with your left hand.

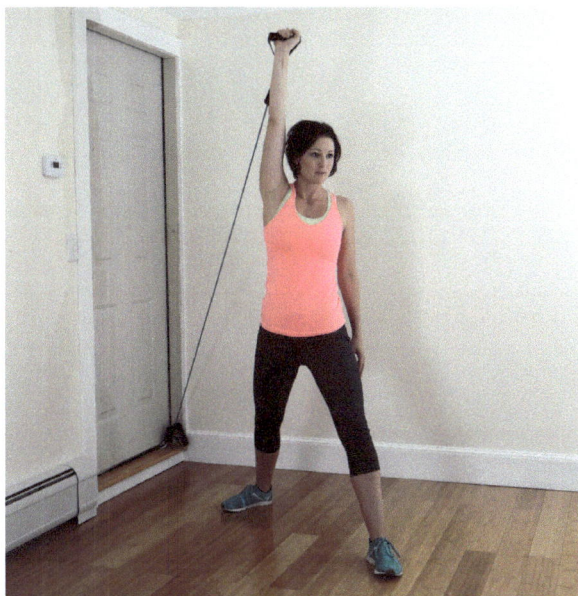

4C.
Press up through your feet and turn to look forward. Maintain the Shoulder Brace and breathe out as you move through the exercise.

"Proper flexibility and mobility is essential to preventing injury."

This series of exercises will help you improve flexibility in your muscles, and mobility with overall movement.

Foam rolling general rules:

1. Do not roll over any joints, other than when we perform mobility exercises along the spine.

2. We are going to divide each major muscle group into three parts: right, left, and middle, focusing on the junction between major muscles.

3. The intention of foam rolling is to break up adhesions that develop both within one muscle and in between different muscles with chronic tightness. These adhesions are difficult to stretch out, but respond very well to the compression and friction generated by the foam roller. Then, we follow the foam rolling protocols with a comprehensive mobility and flexibility program. By following the foam rolling with a stretching routine, we are both breaking up these adhesions as well as stretching them.

4. You may feel some tender spots within each muscle as you foam roll. These are adhesions and indicate areas where you have overworked the muscles.

5. Stop if you feel pain in any joint, especially when we get into the shoulder. This is an indication that there may be an old injury within the joint that may need further evaluation.

A. Lower extremity foam rolling.

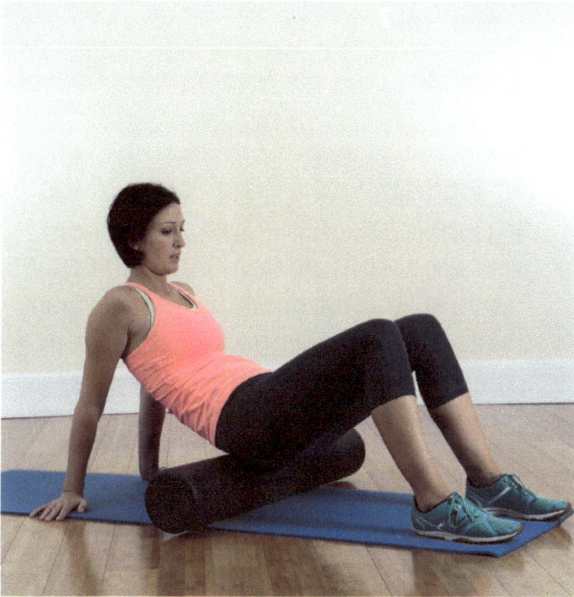

1. Upper glutes and low back. Foam rolling this area will help with hip flexibility, allowing for you to squat deeper and increase your running stride.

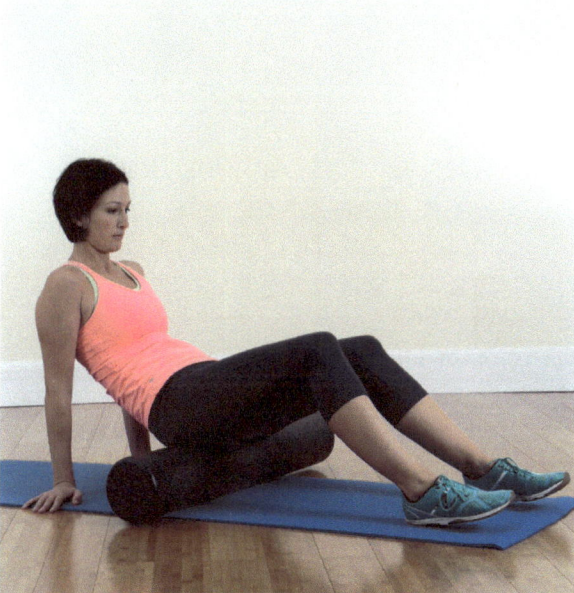

2. Lower glutes and upper hamstrings. This area often gets restricted with years of running or walking. By foam rolling the junction of these two major muscle groups, you will allow both of them to move more freely and improve your mobility.

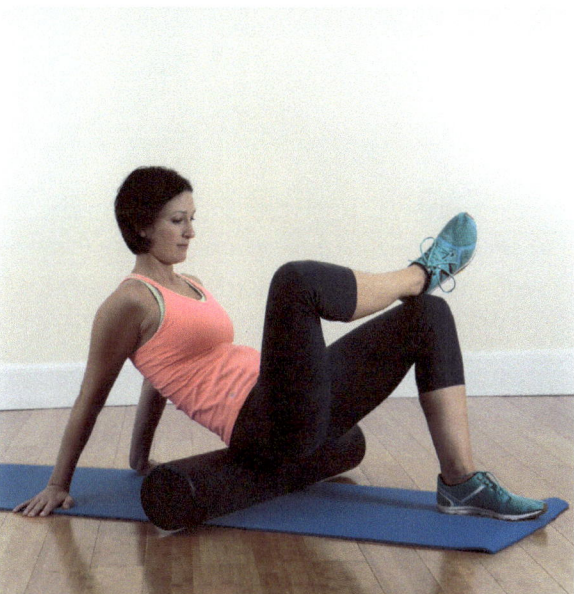

3. Hip rotators, including piriformis. When there is weakness in the gluteus maximus (the biggest of all the glute muscles) and the core, the hip rotators will take over and become overworked. This can result in conditions such as piriformis syndrome.

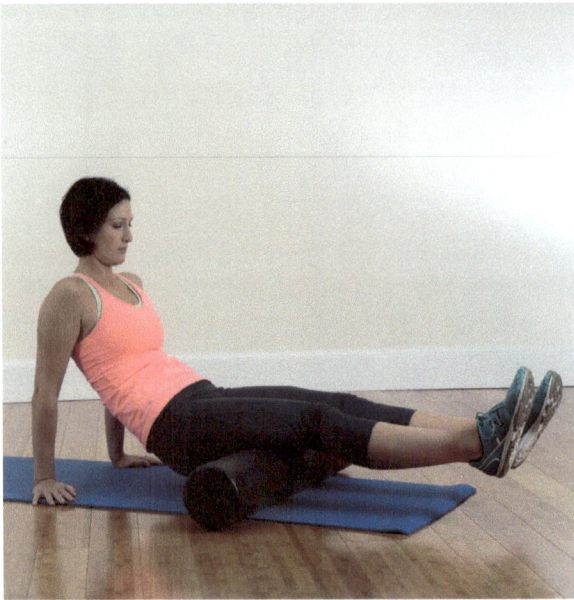

4. Hamstrings. The hamstrings are one of the most commonly overworked muscles in the legs. Flexible hamstrings are essential for everyone, and help with proper squatting, jumping and lunging.

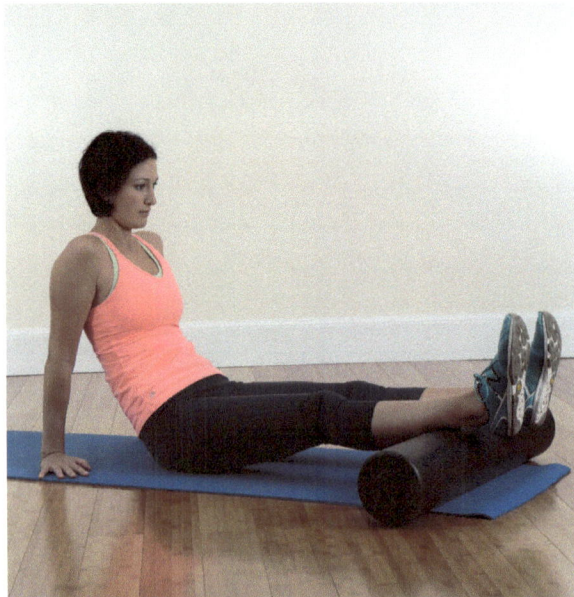

5. Calves and Achilles tendons. Often a focus of runners, the calf muscles can become chronically restricted with previous conditions such as previous ankle sprains, wearing heels every day, or plantar fasciitis.

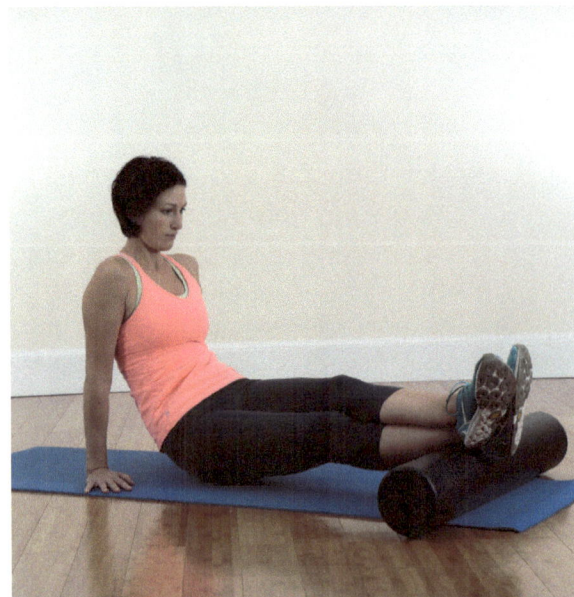

6. Intensive and isolated calf. By placing one leg over the other, this will add pressure to the calf and Achilles, providing a more isolated treatment of each muscle.

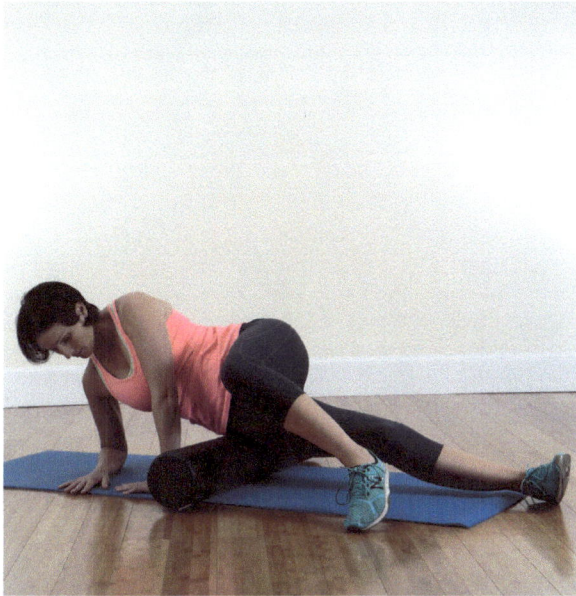

7. TFL and IT band (lateral hip and knee stabilizers). The TFL is the muscle at the top of the IT band. This is often restricted with IT band syndrome, a common repetitive use injury of runners.

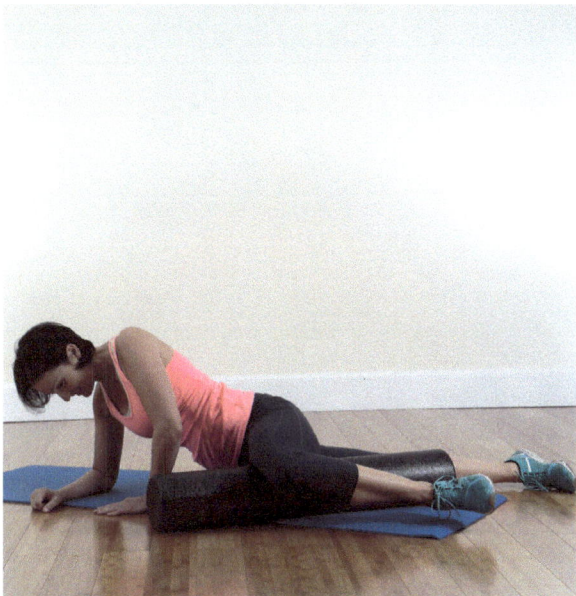

8. Adductors (the inner thigh). These muscles often get overworked with repetitive use and can contribute to hip or knee pain.

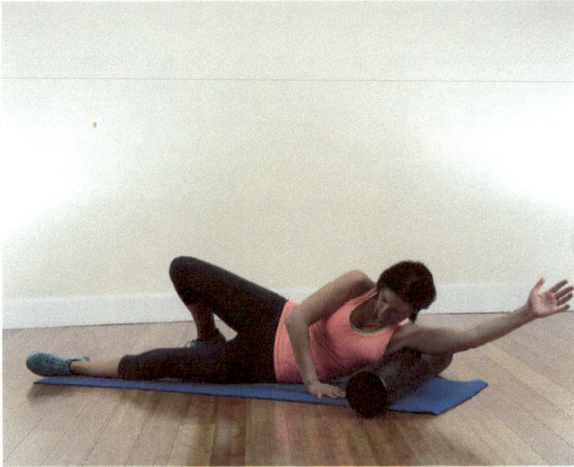

1. Latissimus dorsi and shoulder rotators. These muscles often get overworked in swimmers and overhead athletes such as tennis players, volleyball players and power lifters.

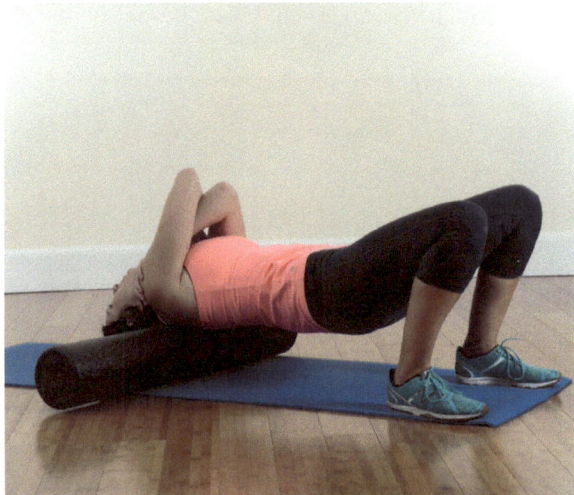

2a. Cross your arms in front of you, place the foam roller in between your shoulder blades. Extend your head and neck.

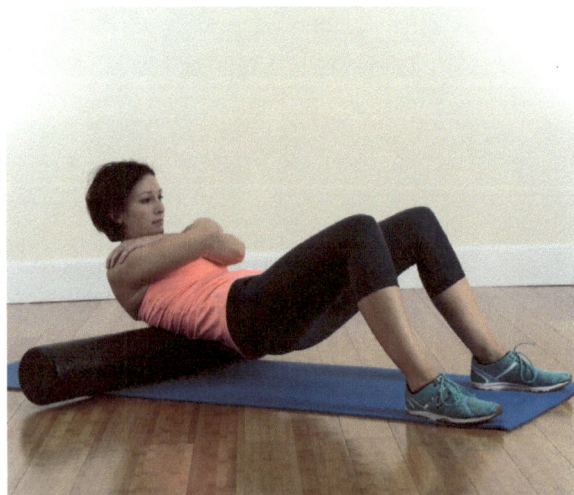

2b. As you roll the foam roller down your back, lift up into a crunch while you stabilize yourself with your feet and hips. This promotes upper back extension, which will help alleviate neck pain and improve mobility throughout the shoulders.

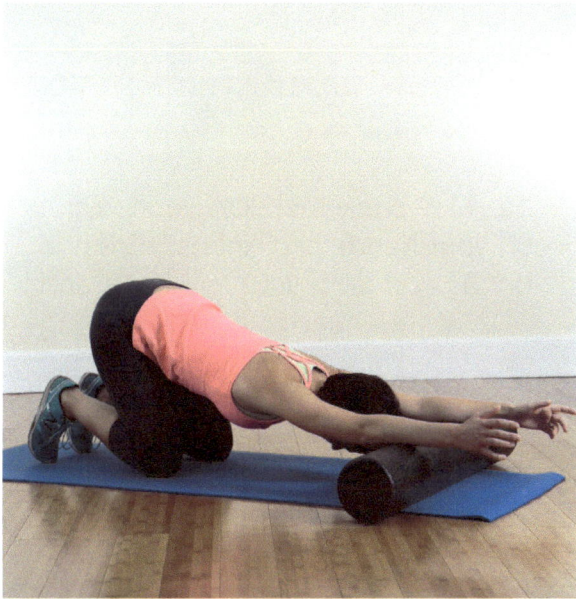

3. This mobility exercise will further promote flexibility and mobility throughout the shoulders and upper back. Be careful, though. If you have pain in the top of your shoulder with this exercise, it may be an indication of a more complicated shoulder problem. In that case, seek professional care. Start in this position with your arms on the foam roller and allow your head and upper back to sink towards the floor.

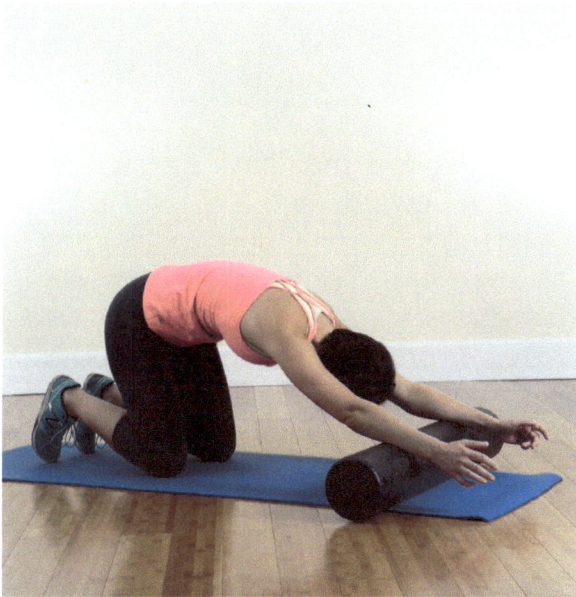

4a. This position transitions into a mobility exercise. Arch your back while maintaining contact with the foam roller. Breathe in as you arch up.

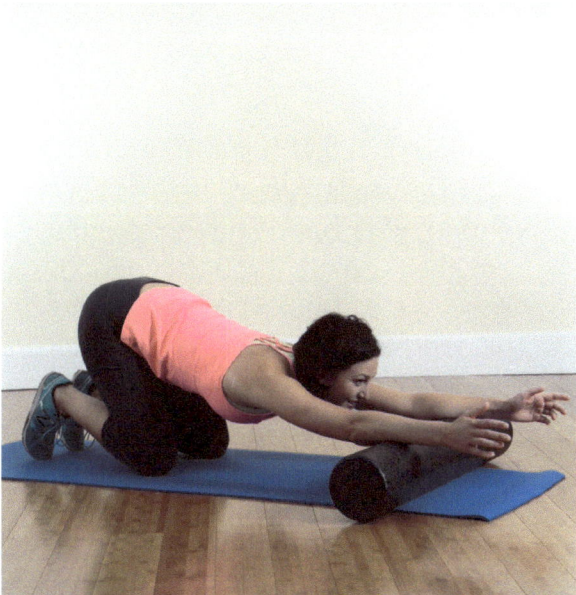

4b. As you breathe out, allow your chest to sink towards the floor and your head to extend. You will feel a stretch throughout your shoulders and back.

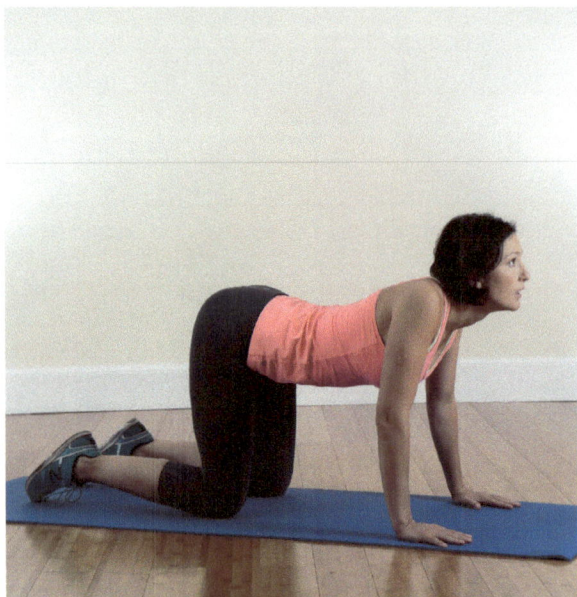

1a. Mid back mobility work. Start on your hands and knees. Breathe out as you arch your low back and extend your head and neck, looking up at the ceiling.

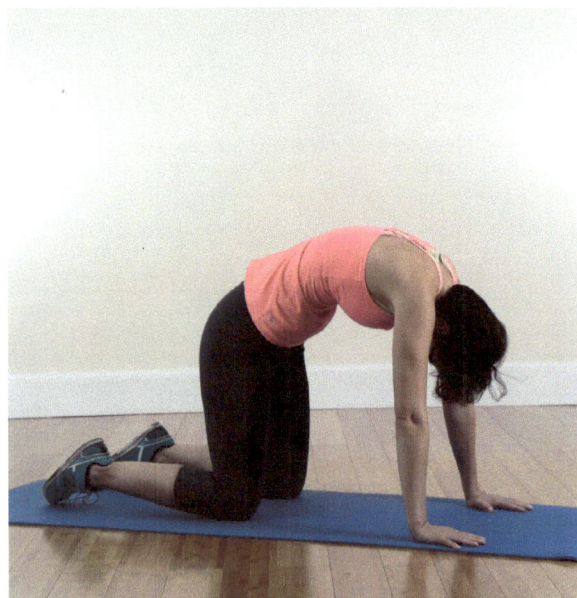

1b. As you breathe in, arch your back upwards and feel the stretch throughout your low back and shoulders. Upper back mobility exercises, such as this, will help promote proper shoulder movement and minimize injuries to the shoulder.

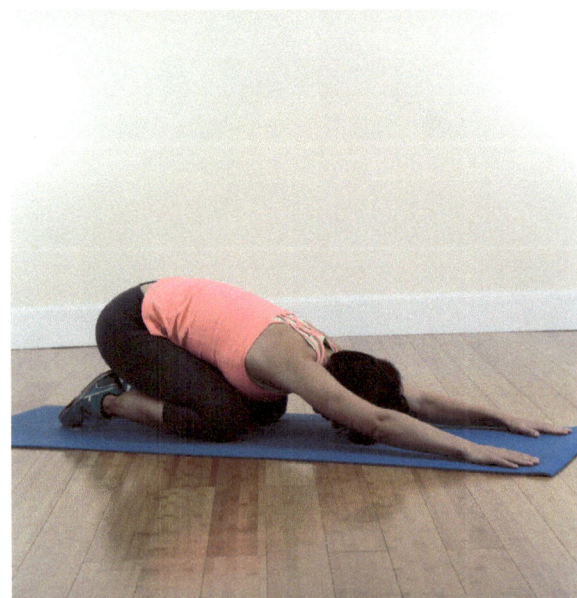

2. Elongated low back stretch. Sit back towards your heels while keeping your hands flat on the mat. Feel the stretch through your low back, upper back, and shoulders. This long stretch addresses the big muscles that cover your entire back.

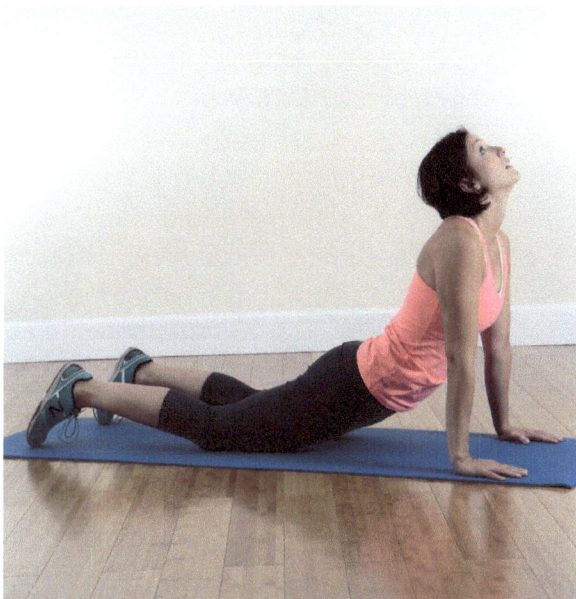

3. Low back extension. As you breathe out, let your hips sink down towards the mat. Keep your shoulder muscles engaged to protect your shoulders and neck. This exercise will stretch the front of your hips and maintain mobility throughout your low back.

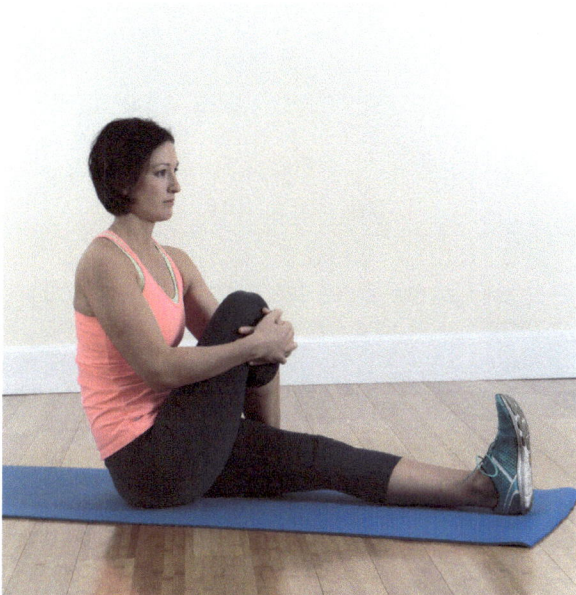

4. Hip rotator stretch. Start seated with your back straight. Cross your right leg over your left leg, hugging your knee to your chest. Pull your right knee towards your left shoulder. The hip rotator muscles live deep in the back of your hip. They often become overworked trying to provide stability to the hip, low back, and even the knee. Even without pain, these muscles are used every day! Take care of them! Reverse to stretch opposite side.

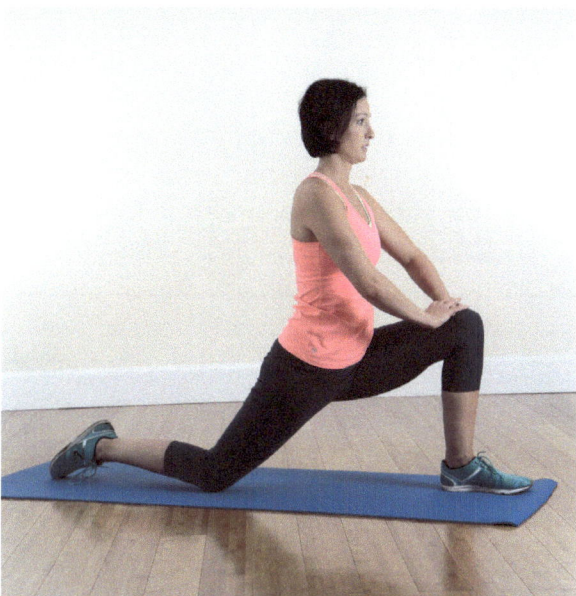

5. Hip flexor stretch. Start in a kneeling position with your right knee back and your left foot placed firmly on the mat. Stay straight and tall through your back and shoulders. Gently, lean forward with your hands placed on your left knee, feeling the stretch in the front of your right hip and thigh. The hip flexor group of muscles is in the front of your hip and into the front of your thigh. This stretch isolates the psoas and iliacus muscles, two of the largest muscles in your body. These can become very short and tight with sitting for prolonged periods of time. Tightness in these muscles can also contribute to low back pain. Reverse to stretch opposite side.

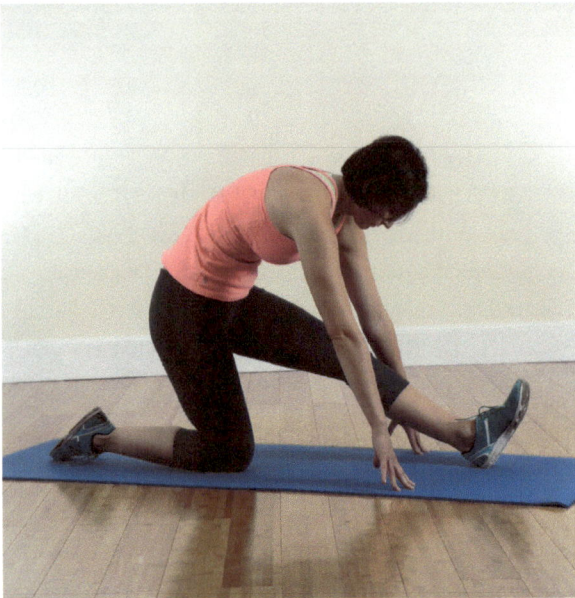

6. Hamstring stretch. Kneel down on your right knee, keeping your left leg straight out in front of you with the heel down on the mat. Using your hands to maintain balance, slowly sit back and bring your right glute towards your right heel. You will feel the stretch in the hamstrings, which are located in the back of your thigh. The hamstrings are worked with running and every day walking. Chronic tightness over time can contribute to knee pain. Reverse to stretch opposite side.

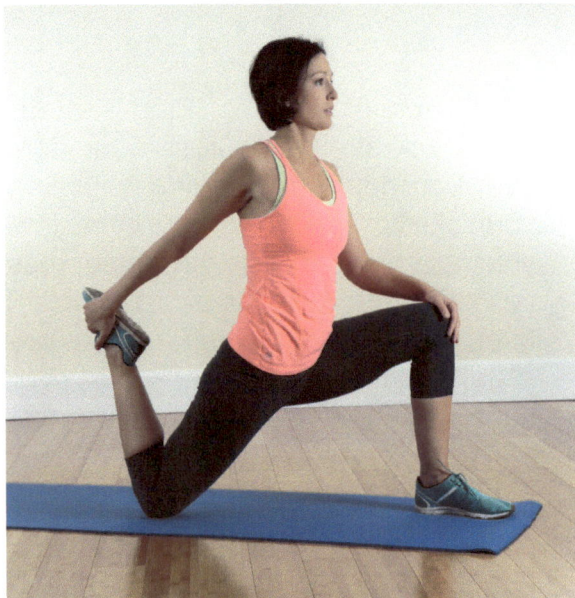

7. Advanced hip flexor, quadriceps, and hamstring stretch. Kneel on your right knee and place your left foot firmly on the mat to create a half-kneeling position. Grab your right foot with your right hand. As you lean forward, also pull your right foot towards your right buttock. Stay tall with this stretch. You will feel the stretch in the right quadriceps (front of the thigh) and hip flexor, and in the left leg hamstring. This stretch targets major muscle groups that move the hip and knee. Reverse to stretch opposite side.

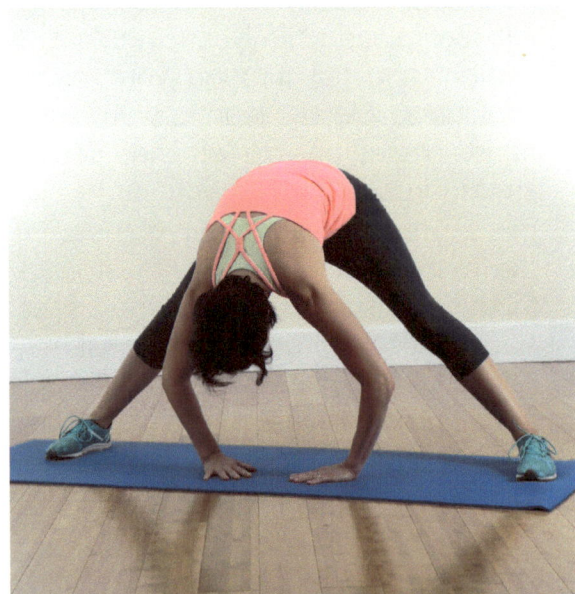

8. Advanced hamstring and low back stretch. Keeping your feet flat on the floor, slowly bend forward to touch the floor. Bring your head towards the floor as far as you comfortably can. Keep your knees straight, but not locked. You will feel the long stretch from the back of your heels to the top of your hips.

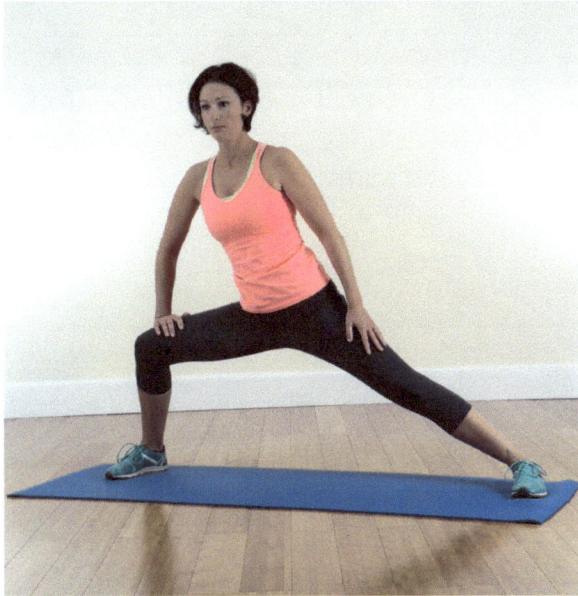

9. From the hamstring stretch above, bend one knee to stretch the adductor group (the groin group) of muscles. Stay tall and don't let your torso "collapse." You will continue to feel a stretch in the hamstring of the bent leg as well. Reverse to stretch opposite side.

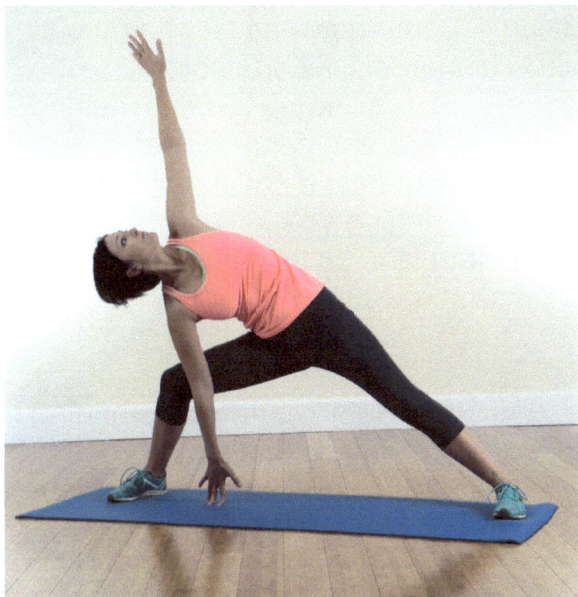

10. From the adductor stretch above, turn your upper body and drop your right hand to the floor. Raise your opposite arm above your head and turn to look at your top hand. This will stretch the whole left side of your body. Reverse to stretch opposite side.

Congratulations! You've completed *Module 2: Restore*. You have retrained your movement patterns to move correctly. Now, you are ready to move more! Keep the party going with high-intensity, short-duration workouts in *Module 3: Excel*.

"Whatever it is, it is possible."

This series of exercises applies the skills and stability learned in Restore and Rebuild to a high intensity, short duration training program.

Module 3: Excel has two levels of progression. Each level has a set of six exercises that should be performed successively. Each set should be repeated three times at least four times per week. You may also incorporate the *Module 2.1.1: Flexibility and Mobility* on the "off days" or on the same day as the workouts.

Module 3.1

1. Squat series - jump squat

A. Intention: The jump squat is a classic exercise. The previous modules have prepared you in both stability, flexibility, and strength. This exercise is a ballistic exercise that requires not only explosive force with high muscle recruitment, but also control of those movements that require the small, stabilizing muscles to be working as well.

B. Description: Begin standing in the squat stance, with feet a little further than shoulder width apart, and feet pointed forward. Squat down as far as you can while maintaining proper form (knees behind your toes, shins perpendicular to the floor, arms behind you, back straight). As you squat down, swing your arm behind you, "locking in" your stability with your feet, shoulders, and core. Disperse your weight evenly throughout your feet and at the bottom of you squat, explode up towards the ceiling, jumping off the ground and swinging your arms to the front of you. As you land, land as softly as possible, and land on the ball of your foot. Without stopping, squat down again, and jump up towards the ceiling. Repeat 10 times.

C. Common mistakes: Many people are concerned with jump squats hurting their knees. By landing softly, this requires the muscles surrounding the knee to work to protect them. It can actually help prevent knee pain if it is done correctly. Watch that your knees stay behind toes. Land softly and control the movement. Do as many as you can correctly until you can reach the goal repetitions and sets.

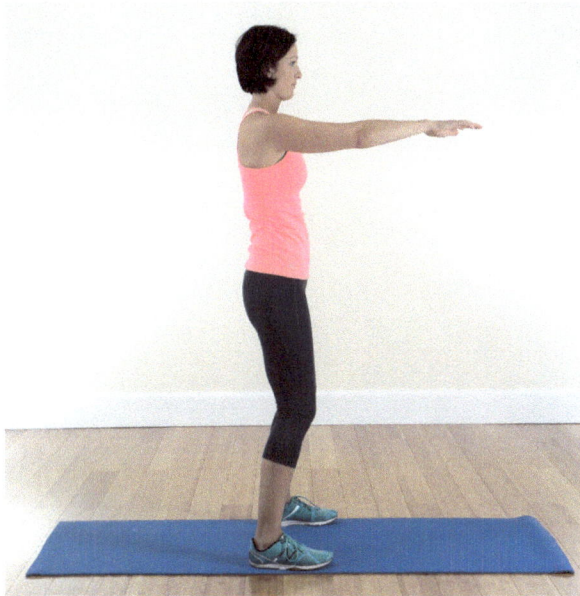

1A.
Start by standing with your feet slightly further than shoulder width apart.

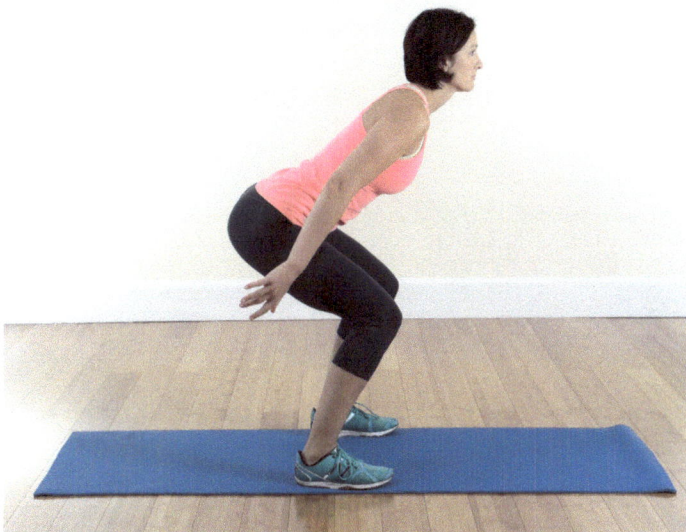

1B.
Bend down, pushing your hips back and keeping your hands to the side.

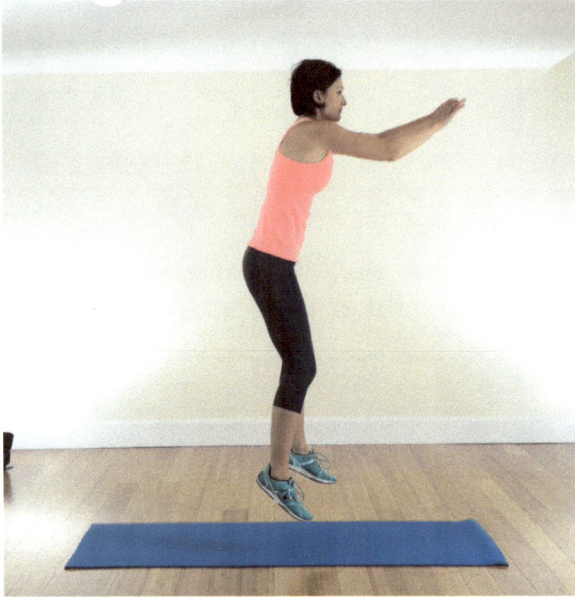

1C.
Spring up, jumping into the air and swinging your arms in front of you.

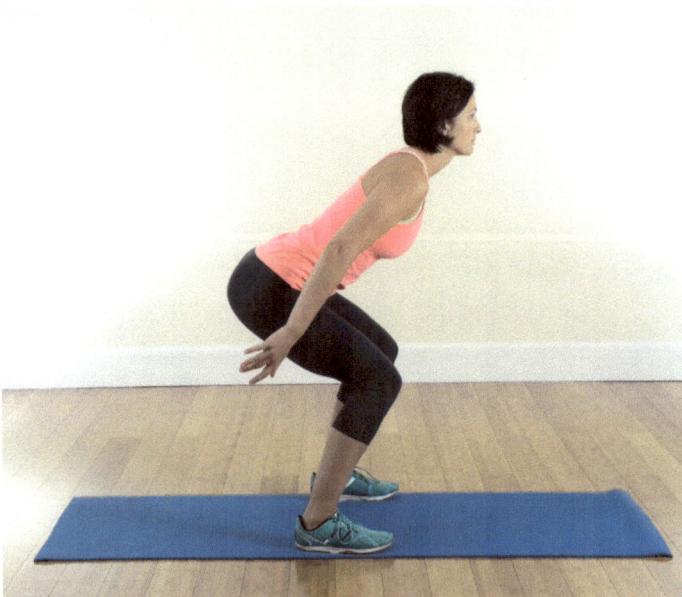

1D.
Land softly and control the movement, moving into a squat as you land. Repeat 10 times.

2. Lunge series – lunge pulse

A. Intention: This exercise works on cross-body stability while requiring flexibility in your shoulders and hips. It will strengthen the bigger muscles, such as the quad (front of your thigh), hamstrings (back of your thigh), hips, and shoulders. This exercise also improves balance.

B. Description: Begin standing with feet shoulder width apart. Perform a PreTrain Brace. Keeping your arms to the side, perform a Shoulder Brace to keep your upper back muscles engaged. Step your right leg in front of you, bending the back left knee to get as close to the floor as possible. The right leg will also bend and make sure to keep your right knee behind your toe. As you step forward with your right leg, bring your arms straight above your head. Focus on two things: contracting both the front and back buttock muscle as you press up, noting the stretch in the front of the hip in your back leg, and pulling your arms up with the muscles in your upper back. Your arms should rise effortlessly as you use your shoulder and upper back muscles. If you feel yourself wobble and your balance challenged, make sure you are fully embracing your PreTrain Brace. Stay in this position, "pulsing" three times each side. Repeat 5 times each leg, alternating legs each time.

C. Common mistake: This is a very challenging exercise and your legs will get tired! Watch that your front knee stays behind your front toe and remember to keep the neck soft. Maintain PreTrain Brace and Shoulder Brace, and focus on contracting the glute muscle in both the front and back leg. Do not be afraid to rest and reset your form.

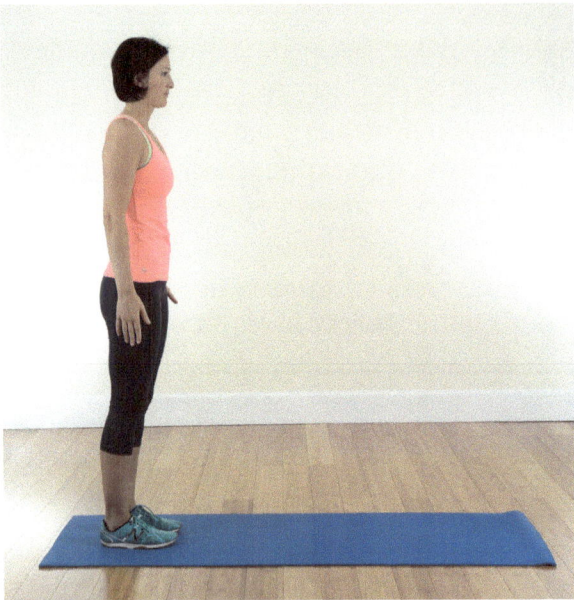

2A.
Start by standing with a neutral spine.

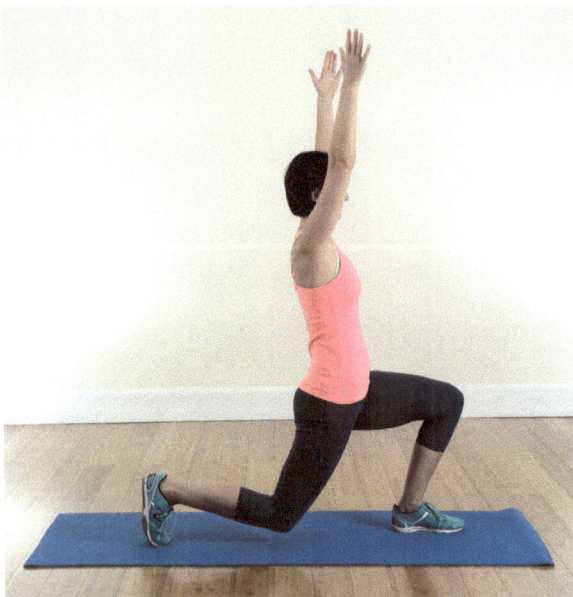

2B.
Step forward with your left leg and engage your Shoulder Brace as you lift your arms over your head. Maintain tension in your back glute.

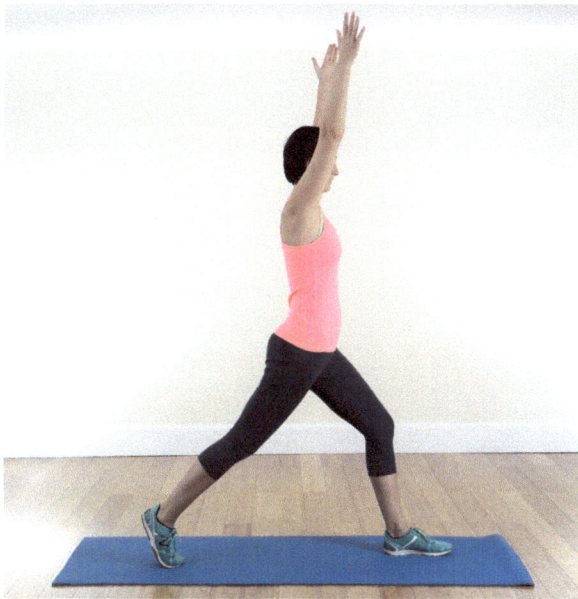

2C.
Keeping the same position with your feet, press up through your feet and legs, feeling all your muscles in your legs engage.

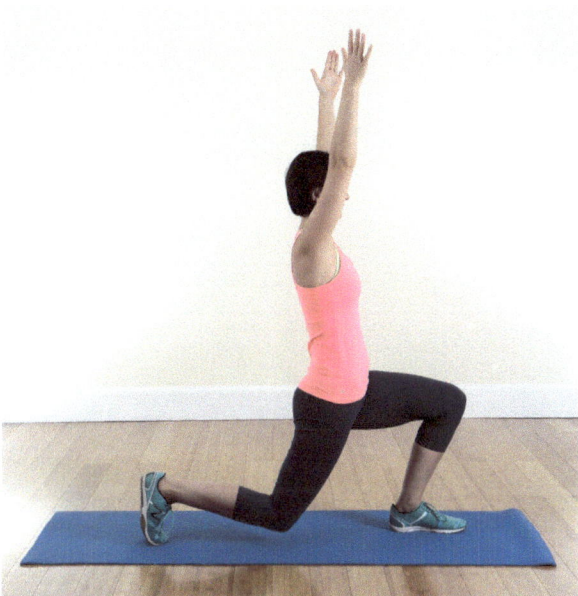

2D.
Return to a lunge position without moving your feet position. Repeat 10 times.

3. Deadlift series - Deadlift with Bosu

A. Intention: This dead lift begins to build strength, while requiring flexibility and mobility. Focusing on strengthening the posterior chain, the biggest muscles in your body, will improve your power, your ability to burn calories, and protect your back.

B. Description: Stand with your feet about shoulder width apart and your feet pointing forward. Place the Bosu ball with the ball side on the floor. "Lock in" the stability with the Lower Extremity Brace. Perform a regular deadlift by hinging your hips behind you, bending at the knees, and keeping your back straight with your core and shoulders engaged. Think about "sinking" back into your hips. Grab the handles of the Bosu ball. This will serve as a counterweight. Perform a PreTrain Brace and exhale as you push your hips forward, pressing your feet into the ground, and lifting your torso upright without moving your spine. Your legs will straighten at the same time, and you will lift the Bosu ball in towards your chest to perform an upright row. Move slowly and tighten your buttocks (glutes) as you lift your torso up, remember to keep your Shoulder Brace engaged. You will feel the strength in between your shoulder blades. Repeat 10 times.

C. Common mistakes: The most common problem is maintaining a straight back. Make sure to keep your shoulders engaged and be careful not to let your low back collapse. If your shoulders are not engaged, your arms will just hang. If you notice this, reset your stability with the PreTrain Brace and Shoulder Brace.

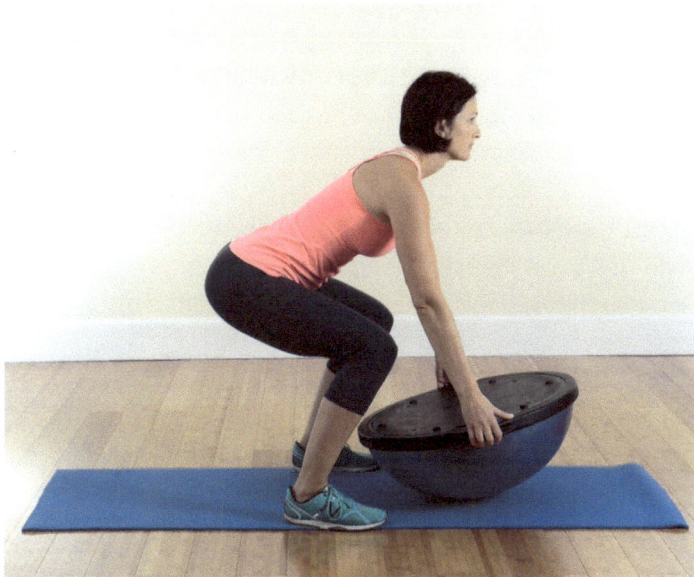

3A.
Begin with feet slightly wider than shoulder width apart. Push your hips back and grab the Bosu ball. Engage PreTrain Brace and Shoulder Brace.

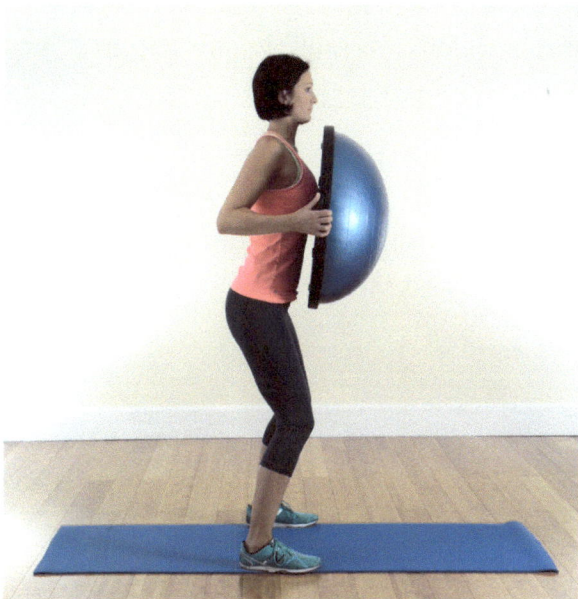

3B.
Press up through your feet and legs, contracting your glutes and pulling the Bosu ball into your chest. Feel the muscles engage in your hips and back.

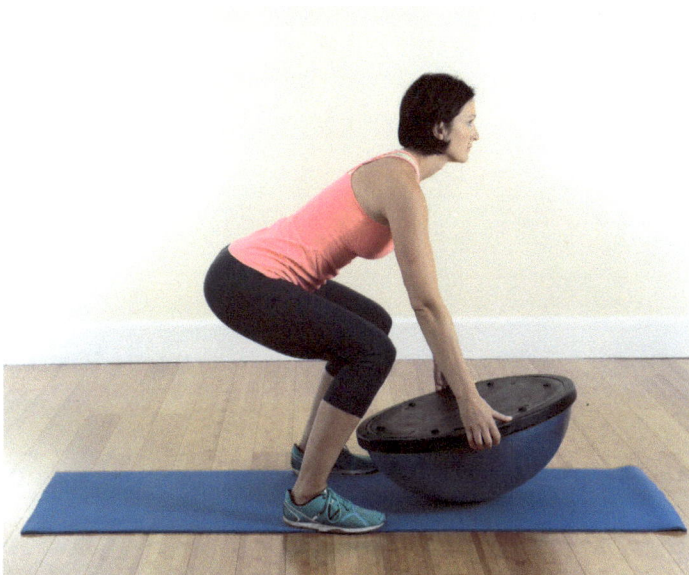

3C.
Return to the starting position with your hips behind you. Maintain tension in your shoulders with the Shoulder Brace.

4. Burpee series - burpee to plank (performed slowly)

The burpee has become a favorite of boot camps, high intensity training, and functional workouts. The burpee combines a plank, a squat, and a squat jump all in one.

A. Intention: The burpee is a great exercise and combines stability, explosive strength, and flexibility. This exercise will get your heart rate up and your muscles burning! It is a great combination of cardiovascular exercise, strength, and stability training.

B. Description: Begin in a standing position with your hands over your head. Drop your butt down and place both hands on the floor a little more than shoulder width apart. Jump your feet back into a plank position and settle into the plank position. Stabilize the shoulders with the Shoulder Brace and keep the PreTrain Brace engaged. Squeeze your glutes and keep your neck neutral. Hold the position in a plank for three seconds. Then, pop your feet forward to the level where your hands were, sitting into a squat, and having your arms in front of you. Think about exploding with your feet underneath you and land into a squat position. Stand up straight. Repeat 10 times, going very slowly and focusing on form.

C. Common mistakes: When the muscles fatigue, the form will first begin to fail in the plank as it requires the most stability. Focus on this movement, and if you begin to feel like you are unable to keep your back straight, slow your movements and focus on the form. Don't be afraid to rest in between repetitions.

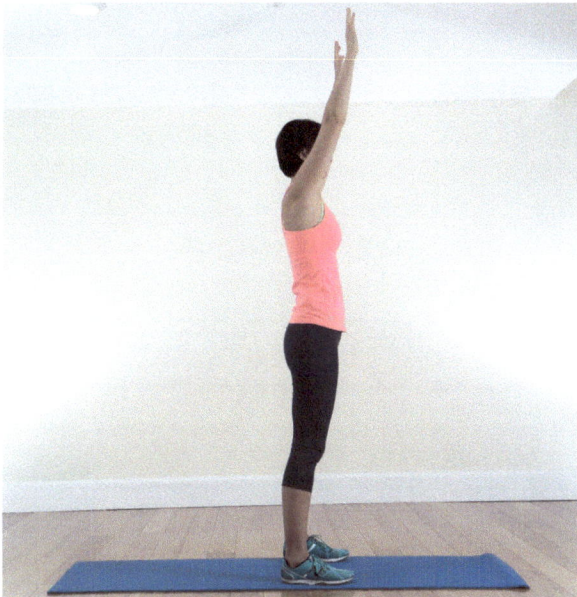

4A.
Start standing with your arms above your head.

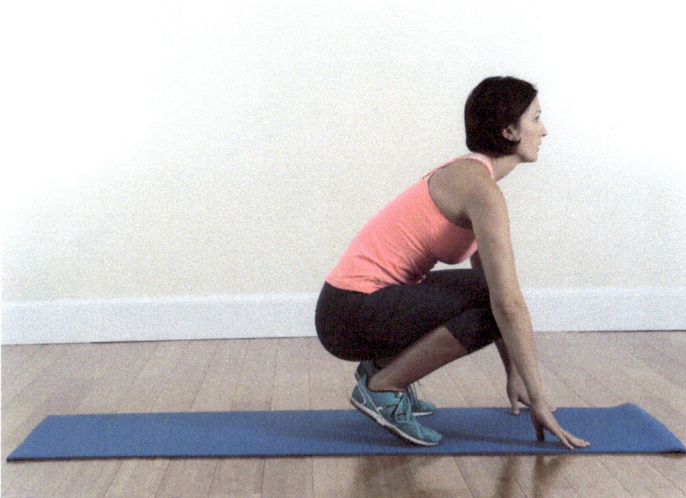

4B.
Squat down with your hands on the floor and your weight on your toes. Keep your back straight.

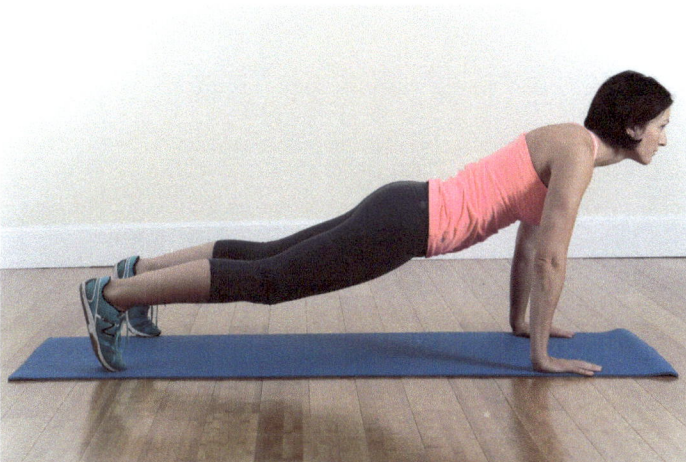

4C.
Spring your feet back into a plank, making sure to engage your PreTrain Brace and Shoulder Brace. Hold the plank for a couple of seconds.

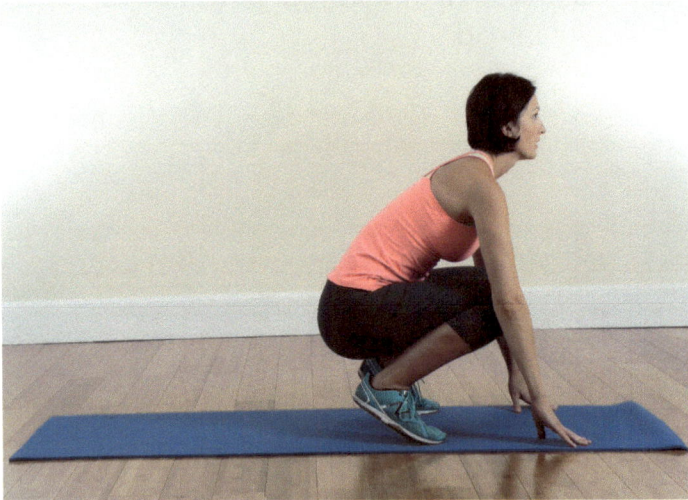

4D.
Jump back into a squatting position.

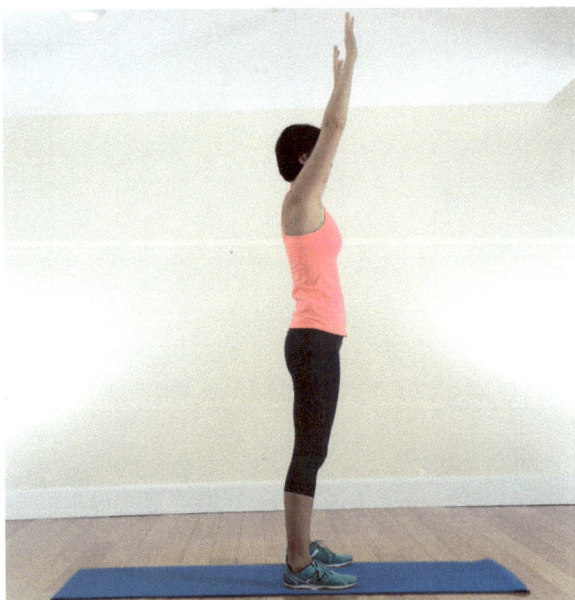

4E.
Return to a standing position.
Repeat 10 times.

5. Push Ups

A. Intention: If done correctly, the push up is a full body exercise. Because your core complex and glutes are engaged, the muscles that are working to move you are building strength and power in the upper body. This exercise maximizes core and shoulder stability with upper back and shoulder strength training.

B. Description: Start on the floor on your hands and knees, with your hands a little further than shoulder width apart. Perform PreTrain Brace and Shoulder Brace. When you feel these stabilizing muscles engage, move from your knees to your toes. Squeeze your buttock muscles to complete a strong and stable plank position. Keep your back straight and your hips stable. Keeping this position, bend your elbows, keeping your head neutral and neck relaxed, lowering yourself to the floor. At the bottom of the push up, press your hands into the floor and think about your mid back muscles, the muscles in between your shoulder blades, pulling you up. Be aware of not letting your hips sag or your neck dip. Repeat 10 times.

C. Common mistakes: Don't let your hips drop and sag as this will put undue stress in your low back. Go as far down to the ground as you can and stop if you feel pain in your shoulder. At this point in the program, you should be able to perform at least one perfect push up. Don't modify the push up. Instead, do as many as you can correctly and focus on building more repetitions from one session to the next.

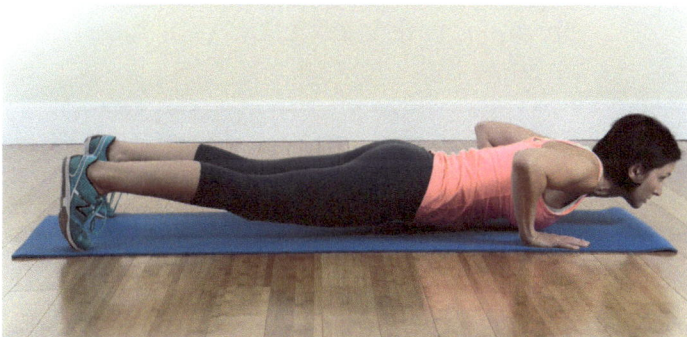

5A.
Begin in a plank position, engaging your PreTrain Brace and Shoulder Brace.

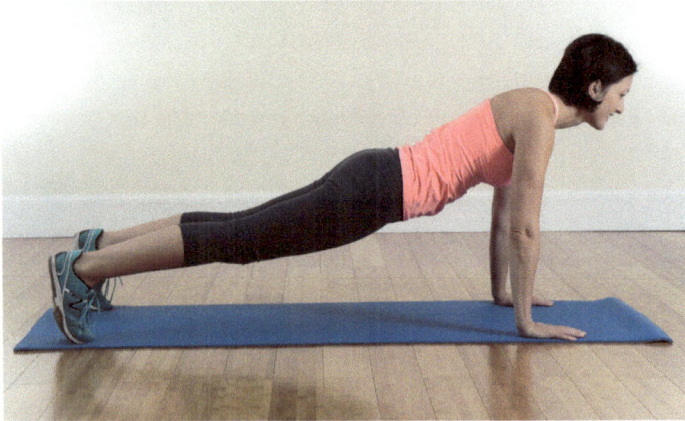

5B.
Keep your shoulders, core, and glutes engaged and lower yourself to the floor, or as close as you can without compromising your form. Press through your hands and use your shoulders and upper back to press up back into a plank position.

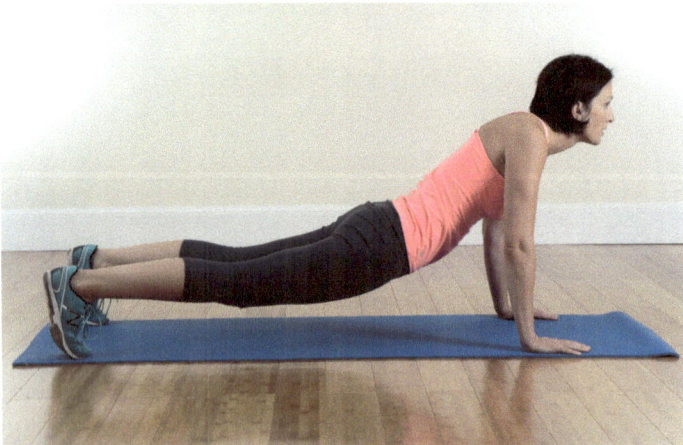

5C.
Common mistake. A common mistake is not engaging the PreTrain Brace and Shoulder Brace properly, which will allow your hips and low back to sag.

6. Plank series - 30 second hold

A. Intention: The plank is typically considered a core exercise. Even though the core is involved, if performed correctly, the plank will work to stabilize the body as a whole, from the shoulders to the core, through the hips and into the lower leg and feet.

B. Description: The plank is the beginning position of the push up. Start on the floor on your hands and knees, with your hands a little further than shoulder width apart. Perform PreTrain Brace and Shoulder Brace. When you feel these stabilizing muscles engage, move from your knees to your toes. Squeeze your buttock muscles to complete a strong and stable plank position. Keep your neck in a neutral position. Hold for 30 seconds.

C. Common mistakes: Do not let your hips sag or your neck strain. Hold the plank as long as you can without compromising form. Work up to holding for 30 seconds.

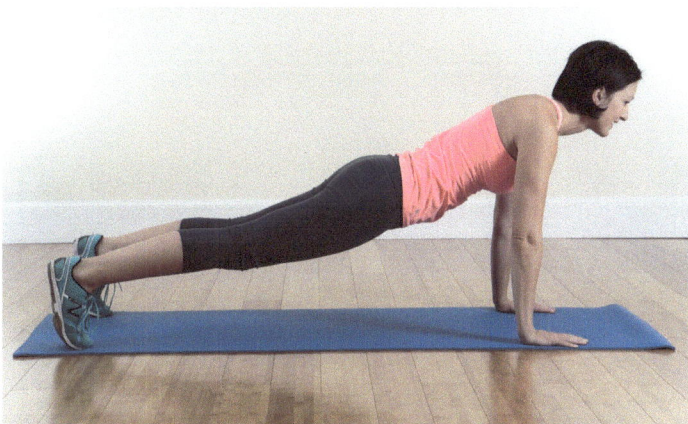

6A. Place your feet and hands slightly wider than shoulder width. Engage the PreTrain Brace and Shoulder Brace. Keep neck relaxed and neutral.

Module 3.2

1. Squat series – Bosu ball squat

A. Intention: The Bosu ball adds a significant stability challenge. This exercise maximizes the challenge of the core from your feet all the way to your shoulders while requiring flexibility in the hips and upper back. This one exercise uses almost every muscle in your body. It will strengthen these muscles, burning fat and building muscle in new areas.

B. Description: Make sure to put the Bosu ball with the flat side on the floor. Carefully step onto the Bosu ball, making sure your feet are approximately shoulder width apart. Start with your arms and hands at your side while you stand on the Bosu ball. Perform the PreTrain Brace and Shoulder Brace, and be aware of the stability in your feet. Slowly, throw your hips back and squat down, making sure your shins stay straight and your knees are behind your feet. Allow your arms to rise in front of you as you squat down. Keeping your braces engaged, drive your feet into the Bosu ball and focus on squeezing your glutes to pull you back into the standing position. Exhale as you stand up. The movements for this exercise are slow and controlled. Move fluidly throughout the movement of the squat, and throughout the 10 repetitions. You should feel the muscles in your foot, lower leg, thigh, hips, and shoulders. There should not be any pain in your back, but you may feel some tension as the deep muscles of the back wall of the core are working.

C. Common mistakes: Be very aware of your form. Do not allow your knees to turn in or turn out too far as this may be an indication of underlying instability. This is a challenging exercise and you will find the exercise getting easier as you move through the repetitions. Squat down only as far as you can without compromising form.

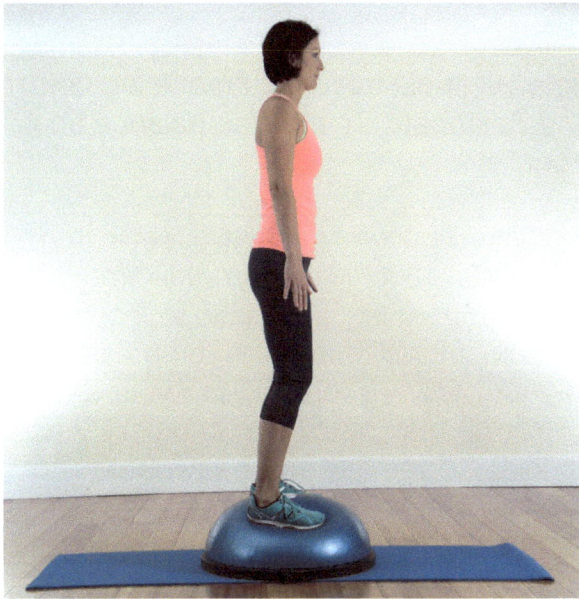

1A.
Start by standing with your feet shoulder width apart on the blue side of the Bosu ball, and your arms to your side. Engage your PreTrain Brace.

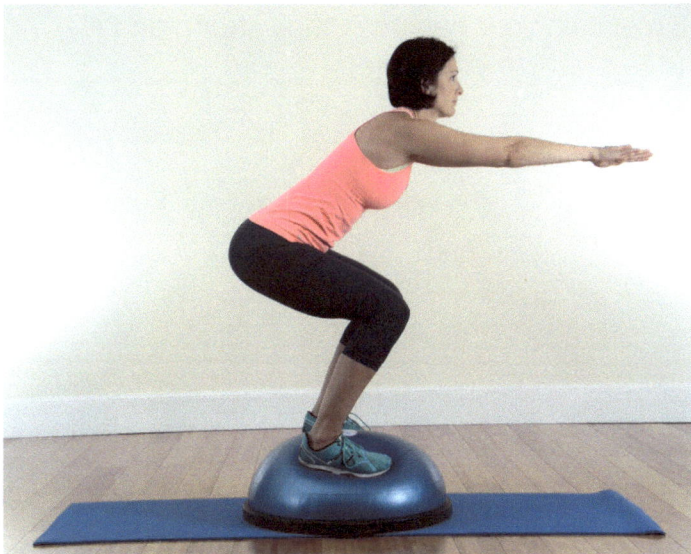

1B.
Squat down, moving your hips behind you and while keeping your knees in line with your toes. Raise your arms in front of you, engaging your shoulder muscles with the Shoulder Brace.

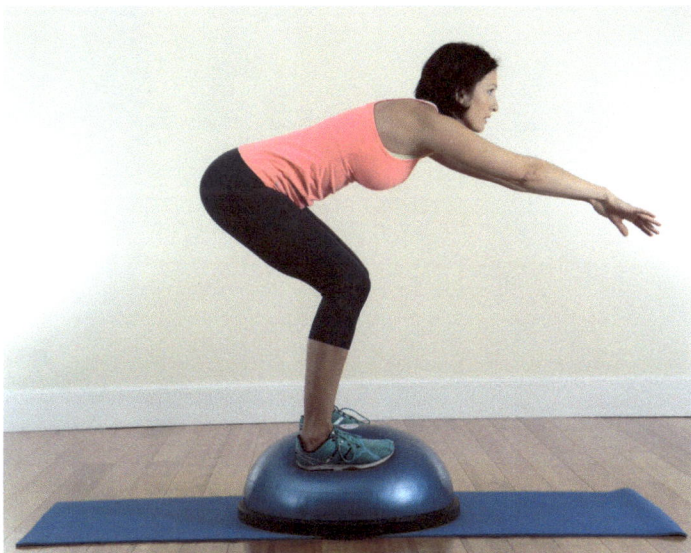

1C.
Common mistake. Be careful not to just bend forward at the waist. To engage your glute muscles, your hips must move behind you to lower your body.

2. Lunge series - lunge on Bosu ball

A. Intention: This exercise increases the challenge of stabilizing on one leg, and maximizes the muscle work with adding the Bosu ball. This builds balance and strength while stretching the hips in the process.

B. Description: Place the Bosu ball, with the flat side down, about two feet in front of you. Perform the lunge as described in Module 3.1. However, this time, as you step forward, step on the Bosu ball with your front leg. Continue to focus on two things: contracting both the front and back buttock muscle as you press up, noting the stretch in the front of the hip in your back leg, and pulling your arms up with the muscles in your upper back. Your arms should rise effortlessly as you use your shoulder and upper back muscles. If you feel yourself wobble and your balance challenged, make sure you are fully embracing your PreTrain Brace. Repeat 10 times each leg.

C. Common mistakes: The Bosu ball will add a significant challenge. The most common difficulty will be maintaining balance throughout the exercise. Focus on the PreTrain Brace as this will help you maintain your balance. Stay strong and if you start to lose your balance, stop and re-stabilize your core.

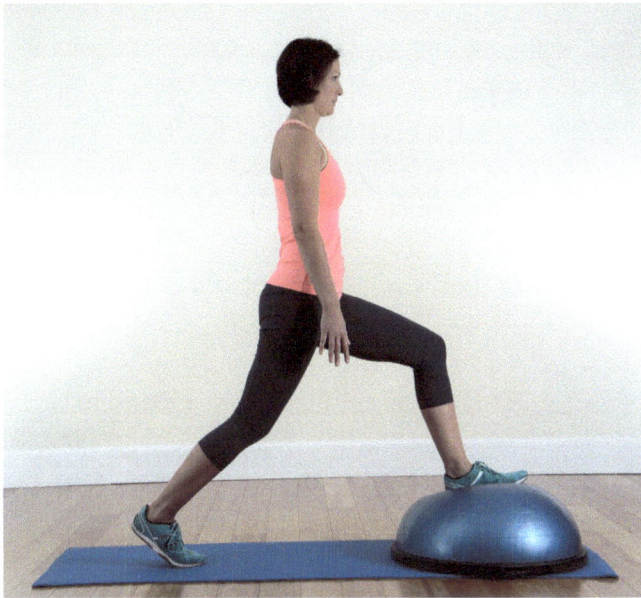

2A.
Start behind the Bosu ball and lunge forward with your left leg. Make sure you have solid contact with the Bosu ball. As you bring your back knee down toward the ground, raise your arms above you. PreTrain and Shoulder Brace are engaged.

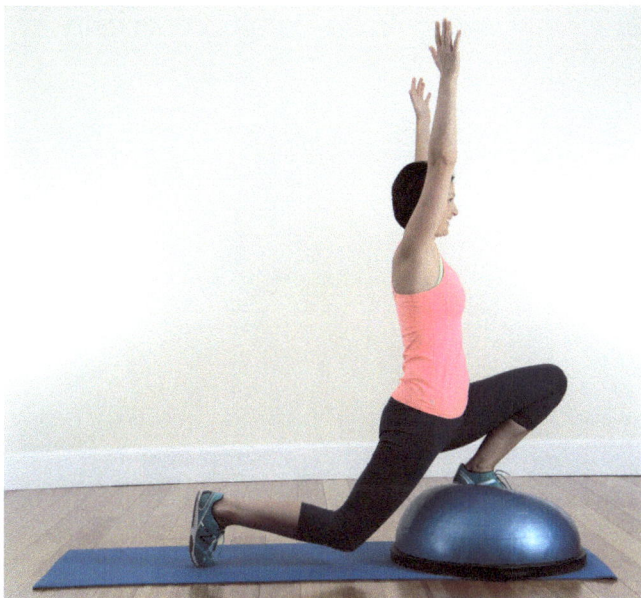

2B.
Common mistake. Be careful not to lose your stability. Do not let your knee go in front of your toes.

3. Deadlift series - deadlift with overhead press

A. Intention: This exercise builds on the Deadlift to include overhead strength training. We are building full body strength with lifting the Bosu ball overhead. This exercise targets the big muscle groups to build muscles fast while challenging the stability of your shoulders and core.

B. Description: Stand with your feet about shoulder width apart and your feet pointing forward. Place the Bosu ball with the ball side on the floor. "Lock in" the stability with the Lower Extremity Brace. Perform a regular deadlift by hinging your hips behind you, bending at the knees, and keeping your back straight with your core and shoulders engaged. Think about "sinking" back into your hips. Grab the handles of the Bosu ball. This will serve as a counterweight. Perform a PreTrain Brace and exhale as you push your hip forward, pressing your feet into the ground, and lifting your torso upright without moving your spine. Your legs will straighten at the same time, and you will lift the Bosu ball in toward your chest to perform an upright row. Move slowly and tighten your buttocks (glutes) as you lift your torso up, remember to keep your Shoulder Brace engaged. You will feel the strength in between your shoulder blades. Move slowly and tighten your buttocks (glutes) as you lift your torso up, raising the Bosu ball over your head. Remember to engage your shoulder stabilizers by bringing your shoulder blades back and down and relaxing the top of your shoulders. Return the Bosu ball to your chest, and then to the floor. Repeat 10 times.

C. Common mistakes: With this exercise, make sure your deadlift form is correct. Be careful not to engage the neck muscles with overhead movement. If you begin to feel strain in your neck, it is an indication that your shoulder stabilizing muscles have become fatigued. Stop and reset the Shoulder Brace before continuing through the exercises.

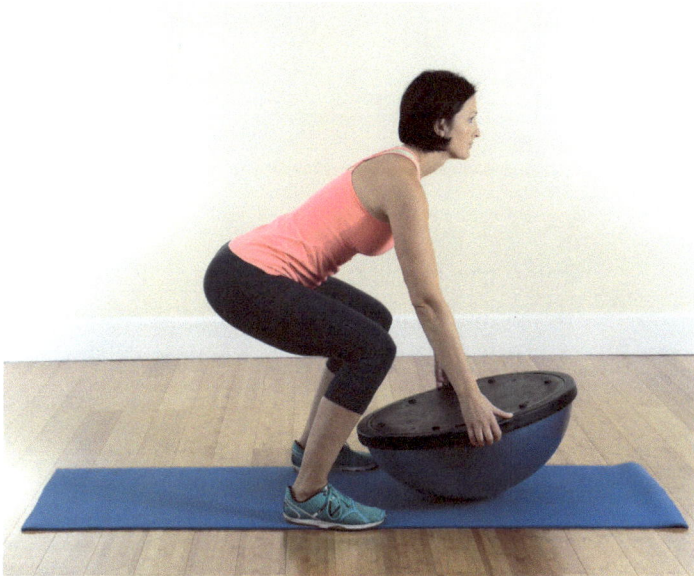

3A.
Begin with your PreTrain Brace, Shoulder Brace, and Lower Extremity Brace engaged. Moving through your hips, sit back into a squat position and grab the Bosu ball.

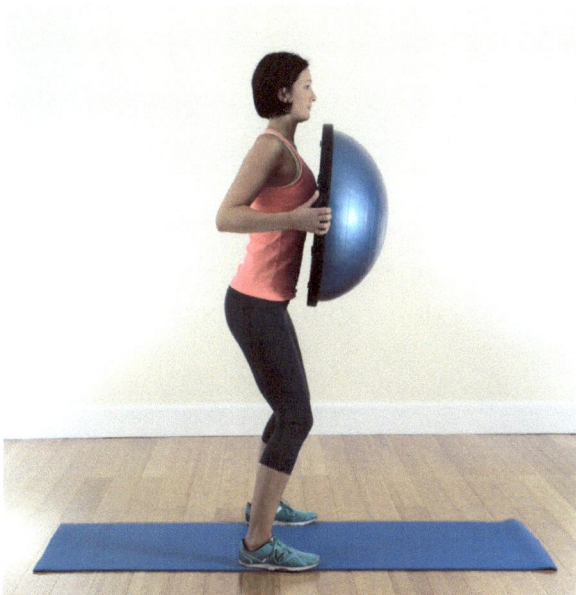

3B.
Press up through your feet, hips, and core to bring the Bosu ball into your chest.

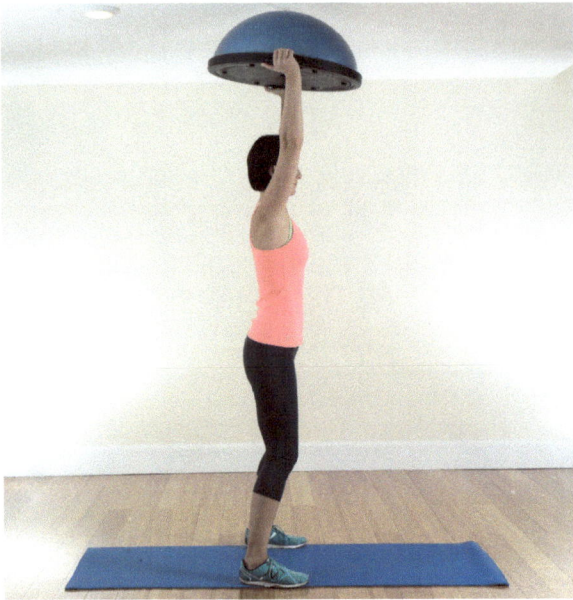

3C.
Raise the Bosu ball overhead. Feel the muscles in your upper back and shoulders engage and stay strong through the movement.

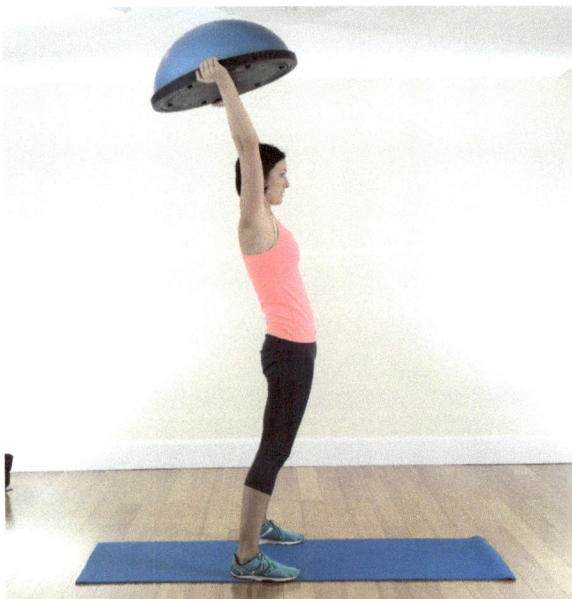

3D.
Common mistake. Be careful not to overextend your low back.

4. Burpee series - burpee to mountain climbers

The burpee has become a favorite of boot camps, high intensity training, and functional workouts. In PreTrain, the burpee will clearly combine a push up, a squat, and a squat jump all in one. This specific exercise will increase your heart rate and challenge your core with the addition of mountain climbers!

A. Intention: This exercise builds on the burpee and incorporates explosive training to build muscle and endurance. This exercise combines stability while building strength in the hips and shoulders while stabilizing the core. Perform each repetition perfectly and don't be afraid to take a break for a minute if you need to catch your breath.

B. Description: Begin in a standing position with your arms over your head. Drop your butt down and place both hands on the floor a little more than shoulder width apart. Jump your feet back into a plank position and settle into the plank position. Stabilize your shoulders using the Shoulder Brace. Keeping your left leg straight and stable and making sure your left glute max is activated, bend your right knee and bring it up in the direction of your right hand. At this point, you should be in a similar position to the one you would be in if you were climbing a mountain (see the connection??:)) except horizontal instead of vertical. After bringing your right knee up, return it to the original position and do the previous step with your left leg. Once again, bend the left knee and bring it up towards the left hand. Perform one more repetition with the right knee forward. Remember to think about engaging the shoulder stabilizers, keeping PreTrain Brace engaged, and squeezing the buttock. Keep the neck neutral. After three repetitions total, explode with your feet underneath you and land into a squat position. Repeat the burpee to mountain climber exercise 10 times, each time, alternating which leg you use initially.

C. Common mistakes: The biggest challenge in this exercise is fatigue. This is a challenging exercise and, as you get tired, your form may begin to be compromised. Stay focused on each individual movement of the burpee, and do not hesitate to rest in between repetitions if you begin to get tired.

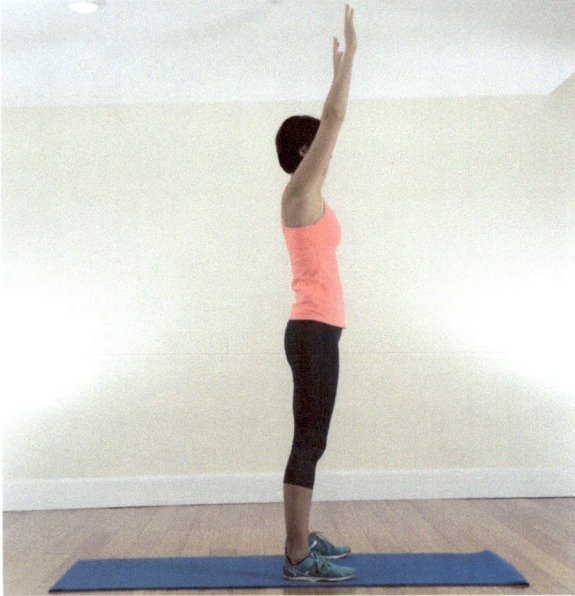

4A.
Start by standing with your arms over your head.

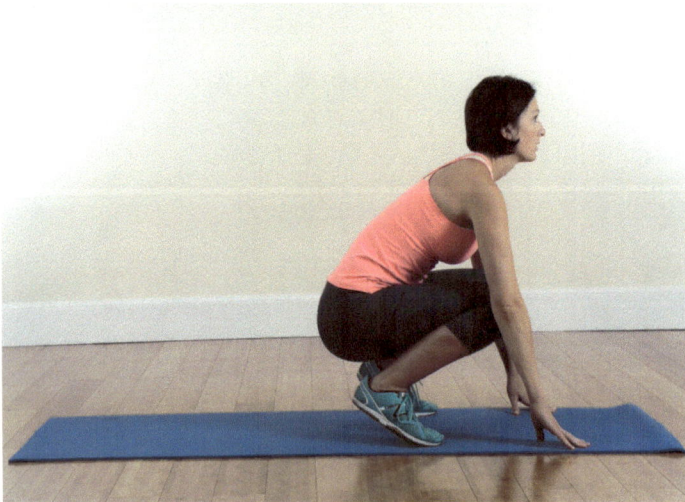

4B.
Squat down so your weight is in your toes. Keep your back straight.

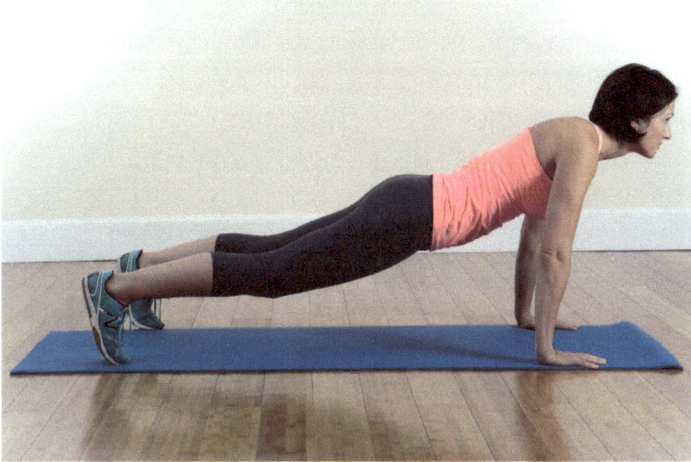

4C.
Jump back into a plank position.

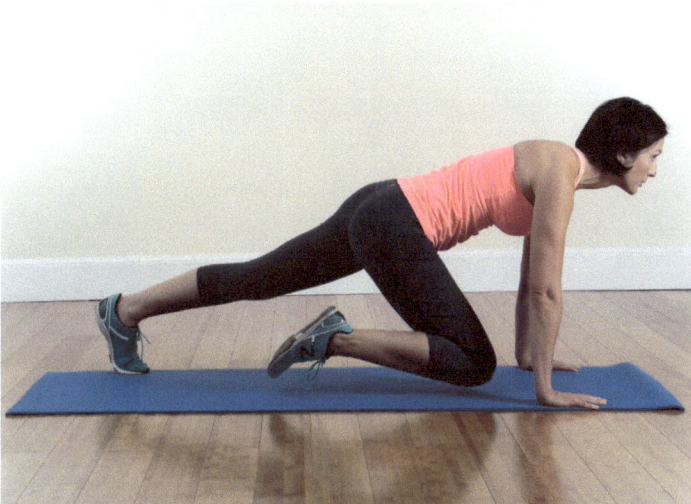

4D.
Maintain stability through your hips, low back, and shoulders. Bring your right knee underneath you. Return back to a plank, and alternate with your left leg and then once more with your right leg. Reverse the series of movements to return back to a standing position.

5. Push up series - push ups on Bosu

A. Intention: The Bosu ball is a unique tool that will allow you to maximize stability with your upper body. This exercise will require almost every muscle in your body. It will build strength in your upper body while maintaining stability in your core and shoulders.

B. Description: Place the Bosu ball with ball side down. Grab each side on the handles of the Bosu ball. Perform PreTrain Brace and Shoulder Brace. When you feel these stabilizing muscles engage, move from your knees to your toes. Squeeze your buttock muscles to complete a strong and stable plank position. Keeping this position, bend your elbows, keeping your head up and neck relaxed, lowering yourself to the floor. At the bottom of the push up, press your hands into the floor and think about your mid back muscles, the muscles in between your shoulder blades, pulling you up. Be aware of not letting your hips sag or your neck dip. Repeat 10 times.

C. Common mistakes: Make sure to keep the neck soft throughout the exercise. There should not be any strain in the neck. If you begin to feel your neck becoming strained, it is an indication that your shoulder stabilizing muscles are fatigued. Also make sure to maintain a proper plank position throughout the push up. Do not let the hips sag.

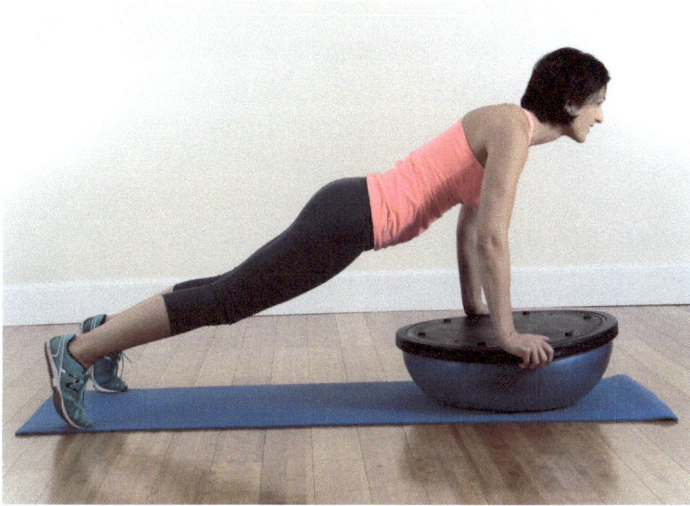

5A.
Begin in a plank position, with your hands on the Bosu ball. Perform a PreTrain Brace and Shoulder Brace. Keep your neck neutral.

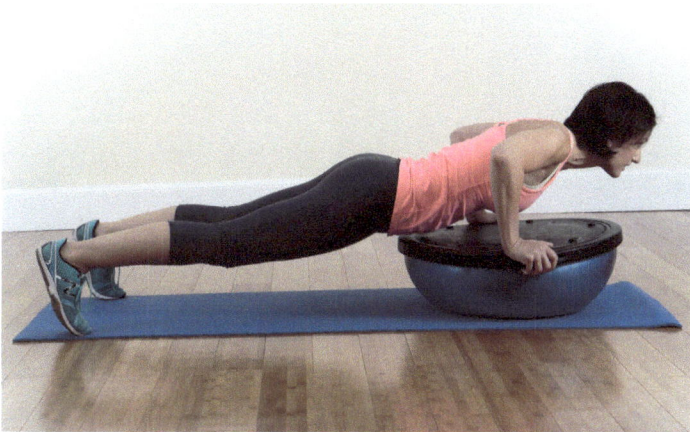

5B.
Lower your body down to the Bosu ball, maintaining stability through your hips and shoulders.

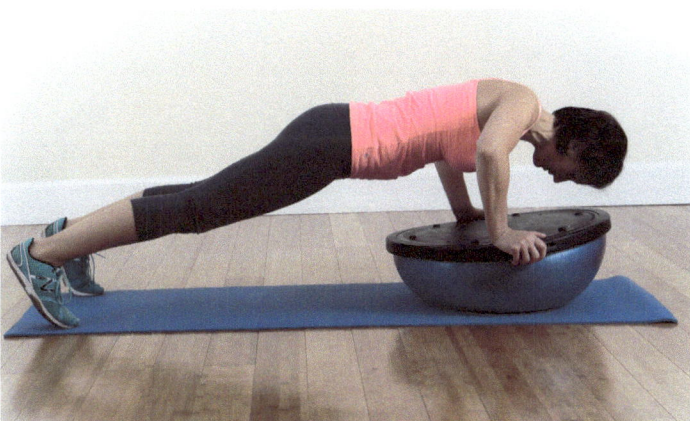

5C.
Common mistake. Be careful not use just move your head down to the Bosu ball. Use your arms and shoulders to lower and raise your body.

6. Plank series - Alternating plank

A. Intention: This is a deceivingly difficult exercise. Holding the plank while transitioning from hand to hand challenges cross body stability. This exercise will strengthen every stabilizing muscle in the upper body and core while building strength in the shoulders, hips, and legs.

B. Description: Start in a plank position. Slowly, with your left shoulder stable and strong turn your body to load your left arm, lifting your right hand to the ceiling so it is in line with your left arm. Keep your feet in the same position, but roll your feet so your torso is in line with your legs and shoulders. Slowly, return your right hand down to the floor, keeping your torso straight and stable, engaging your Shoulder Brace and PreTrain Brace. Hold the plank position for 2-3 seconds. Then, transfer onto your right hand, raising your left hand to the ceiling until it is in line with your right arm. Move slowly and deliberately, holding the PreTrain Brace and Shoulder Brace throughout the exercise. Repeat 10 full repetitions.

C. Common mistakes: The most challenging part of this exercise is maintaining a plank position while transferring from a regular plank to a side plank. To keep the plank stable, make sure to contract the glutes and core.

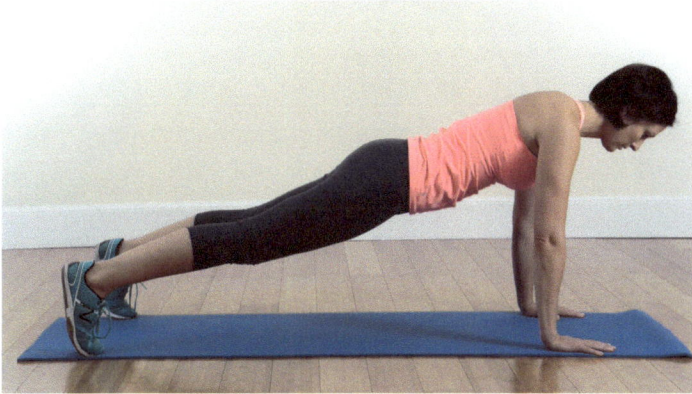

6A.
Begin in a plank position, maintaining your PreTrain Brace and Shoulder Brace with your neck in a neutral position.

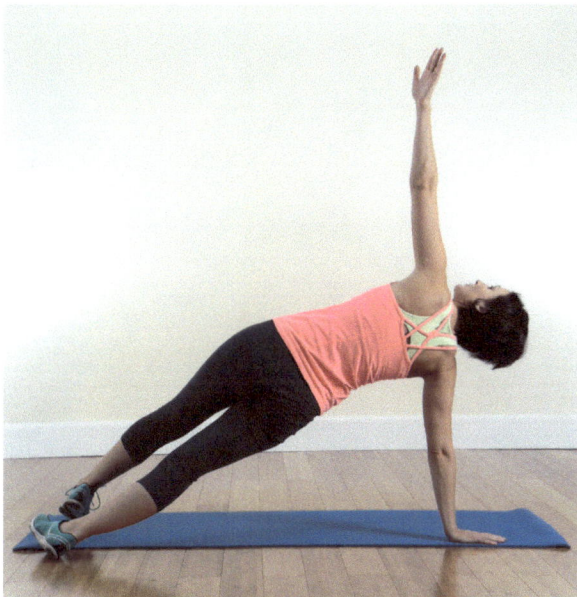

6B.
Rotate your feet and turn your body to raise your left arm above your head. Turn and look at your right hand. Maintain strength and stability throughout your upper body, shoulders, core, and hips.

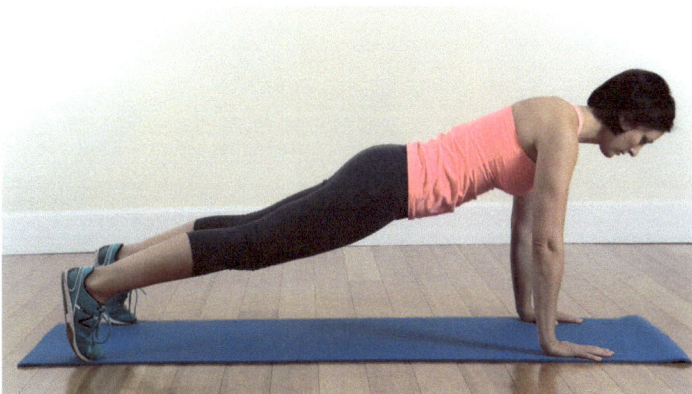

6C.
Return to a plank position.

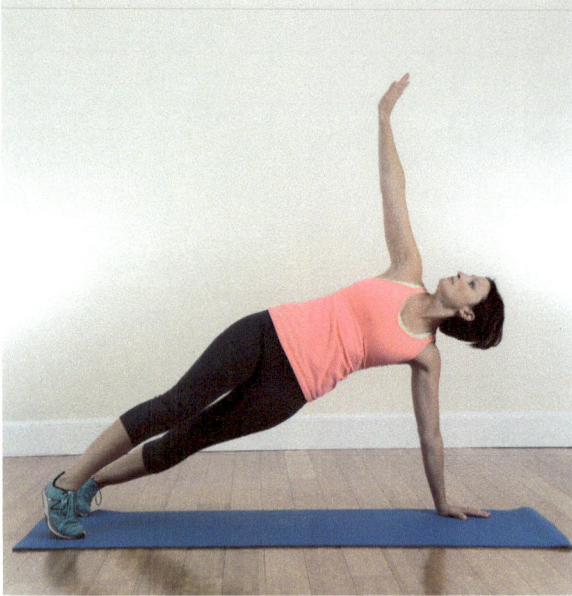

6D.
Alternate to the opposite side.

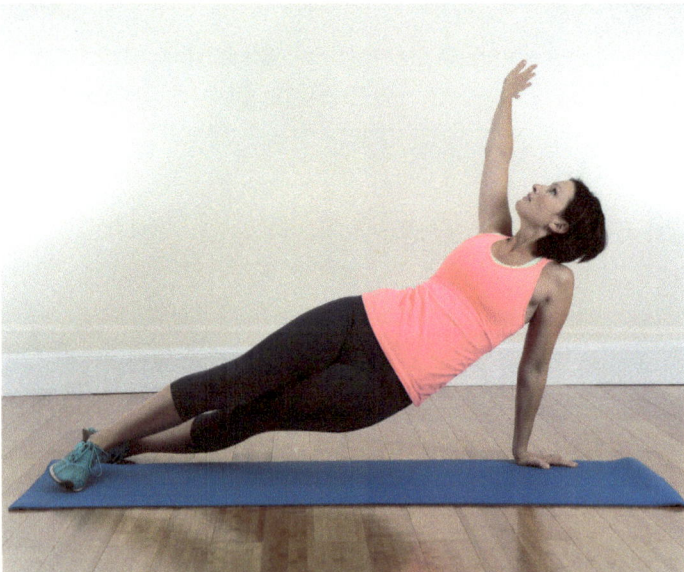

6E.
Common mistake. Be careful not to "swing" your body from side to side. This exercise challenges your full body strength and stability throughout the movement.

Congratulations! You have completed the PreTrain Fundamentals program. You are now moving with improved strength, stability, and mobility. Continue using PreTrain Fundamentals as a maintenance program to maximize the positive effects on training, and on your life.

For more information, visit
www.PreTrain.com

Afterword

Congratulations on completing PreTrain Fundamentals! Now what?

You have worked very hard to get to a stronger, more stable, and more flexible self. The intensive PreTrain Fundamentals program will now serve as a maintenance program. You will see benefits from performing any of the Modules regularly. However, for best results, the recommended maintenance program combines the following modules for an intense, 45 minute workout:

- Module 1.2
- Module 2.2
- Flexibility Module
- Module 3.1 or 3.2

Performing this series of modules once a week will help to maintain the improvements you have made. It will address every muscle, big and small, as well as your flexibility. Remember: the best exercise program addresses the three pillars of fitness: flexibility/mobility, strength, and stability. PreTrain Fundamentals will complement your exercise routine, enhancing your everyday life.

References

1. Cook, G. (2010). Movement: Functional movement systems: Screening, assessment, and corrective strategies. Santa Cruz, CA: On Target Publications.

2. Starrett, K., & Cordoza, G. (2013). Becoming a supple leopard: The ultimate guide to resolving pain, preventing injury, and optimizing athletic performance. Las Vegas, NV: Victory Belt Publishing.

3. Rippetoe, M., & Bradford, S. (2013). Starting strength: Basic barbell training (3rd ed.). Wichita Falls, TX: The Aasgaard Company.